T0324061

Essential CNS Drug Development

Essential CNS Drug Development

Edited by

Amir Kalali
Vice President, Medical and Scientific Services, and Global Therapeutic Team Leader (CNS) at Quintiles Inc, and Professor of Psychiatry at the University of California San Diego, San Diego, CA, USA

Sheldon Preskorn
Professor of Psychiatry, Kansas University School of Medicine-Wichita (KUSM-W), and Chief Science Officer, KUSM-W Clinical Trial Unit, Wichita, KS, USA

Joseph Kwentus
Clinical Professor at the University of Mississippi Medical Center, Jackson, MS, USA

Stephen M. Stahl
Adjunct Professor of Psychiatry at the University of California San Diego, San Diego, CA, USA, and Honorary Senior Visiting Fellow at the University of Cambridge, UK

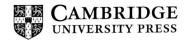

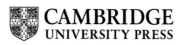

Shaftesbury Road, Cambridge CB2 8EA, United Kingdom

One Liberty Plaza, 20th Floor, New York, NY 10006, USA

477 Williamstown Road, Port Melbourne, VIC 3207, Australia

314–321, 3rd Floor, Plot 3, Splendor Forum, Jasola District Centre, New Delhi – 110025, India

103 Penang Road, #05–06/07, Visioncrest Commercial, Singapore 238467

Cambridge University Press is part of Cambridge University Press & Assessment, a department of the University of Cambridge.

We share the University's mission to contribute to society through the pursuit of education, learning and research at the highest international levels of excellence.

www.cambridge.org
Information on this title: www.cambridge.org/9780521766067

© Cambridge University Press & Assessment 2012

First published 2012
Reprinted 2012

A catalogue record for this publication is available from the British Library

Library of Congress Cataloging-in-Publication data
Essential CNS drug development / edited by Amir Kalali . . . [et al.].
      p.   cm.
   Includes bibliographical references and index.
   ISBN 978-0-521-76606-7 (Hardback)
   I. Kalali, Amir.
   [DNLM: 1. Central Nervous System Agents–pharmacology. 2. Clinical Trials as Topic–methods. 3. Drug Evaluation–methods. 4. Drug Evaluation, Preclinical–methods. QV 76.5]
   615.1´9–dc23

                                                                      2011046215

ISBN   978-0-521-76606-7   Hardback

....

Contents

Contributors

Leslie Citrome, MD, MPH
Clinical Professor of Psychiatry &
Behavioral Sciences, New York
Medical College, Valhalla, NY, USA

Alan J. Cross, PhD
Chief Scientist CNS & Pain Innovative
Medicines Unit, AstraZeneca Research &
Discovery, Wilmington, DE, USA

Judith Dunn, PhD
CNS Site Head, Product Development,
Roche Inc., Nutley, NJ, USA

Kenneth R. Evans, PhD
President and CEO, Ontario Cancer
Biomarker Network, MaRS Centre,
Toronto, Canada

Douglas E. Feltner, MD
Adjunct Clinical Professor, Department of
Psychiatry, University of Michigan, Ann
Arbor, MI, USA

Philip D. Harvey, PhD
University of Miami Miller School of
Medicine, Miami, FL, USA

Amir Kalali, MD
Vice President, Medical and Scientific
Services, and Global Therapeutic
Team Leader (CNS), Quintiles Inc.,
and Professor of Psychiatry, University
of California San Diego, San Diego,
CA, USA

Richard S. E. Keefe, PhD
Duke University Medical Center,
Durham, NC, USA

Michael Krams, MD, PhD
Janssen Pharmaceutical Companies of
Johnson & Johnson, Titusville, NJ, USA

Joseph Kwentus
Clinical Professor at the University of
Mississippi Medical Center, Jackson, MS, USA

Matthew Macaluso, DO
Department of Psychiatry and Behavioral
Sciences, University of Kansas School of
Medicine-Wichita, and KU-Wichita
Clinical Trials Unit, KS, USA

Craig H. Mallinckrodt, PhD
Eli Lilly & Co., Lilly Corporate Center,
Indianapolis, IN, USA

Geert Molenberghs, PhD
I-BioStat, Hasselt University, Diepenbeek,
Belgium, and Katholieke Universiteit
Leuven, Leuven, Belgium

Nuala Murphy, PhD
Vice President and Global Unit Head, CNS
and Internal Medicine, Quintiles, Inc.,
Levallois-Perret, France

Ginette Nachman, MD, PhD
Medical Writing Scientist, Global
Regulatory Affairs and Medical Writing,
Quintiles, Inc.

Sheldon Preskorn, MD
Professor of Psychiatry, Kansas University
School of Medicine, Wichita (KUSM-W),
and Chief Science Officer, KUSM-W
Clinical Trial Unit, Wichita, KS, USA

William R. Prucka, PhD
Eli Lilly & Co., Lilly Corporate Center,
Indianapolis, IN, USA

Penny Randall, MD, MBA
Quintiles, Inc. and Assistant Professor
of Psychiatry, University of California,
San Diego, CA, USA

Frank D. Yocca, PhD
VP and Head, Strategy Unit, CNS & Pain Innovative Medicines Unit, AstraZeneca Research & Discovery, Wilmington, DE, USA

Gwen L. Zornberg, MD, ScD
Contracting Officer Representative, Epidemiology Research Contracts, Team Leader, Regulatory Science Staff, FDA/CDER/Office of Surveillance and Epidemiology, Silver Spring, MD, USA

Preface

It was the best of times, it was the worst of times, it was the age of wisdom, it was the age of foolishness, it was the epoch of belief, it was the epoch of incredulity, it was the season of Light, it was the season of Darkness, it was the spring of hope, it was the winter of despair, we had everything before us, we had nothing before us, we were all going direct to heaven, we were all going direct the other way – in short, the period was so far like the present period, that some of its noisiest authorities insisted on its being received, for good or for evil, in the superlative degree of comparison only.

Charles Dickens
A Tale of Two Cities

Reminiscent of Dickens, the title of our book could also be "A Tale of Two Disciplines." That is, the discipline of clinical trials in the field of central nervous system disorders is now experiencing both the best of times and the worst of times.

The best of times are exemplified by the explosion of genomics and neuroimaging making possible the best translational neuroscience studies in the history of psychiatry and neurology. Findings from preclinical studies can be forward translated into novel, small population studies in well defined patient groups, utilizing powerful new technologies, and then these results backtranslated to inform better preclinical studies. Never before have the prospects been so great for gaining an understanding of the biological basis of psychiatric and neurological disorders. This might be our age of wisdom, our season of life, our epoch of belief and our spring of hope.

Alas, it is also the worst of times, as shown by the inflating placebo response rate worldwide, destroying our ability to prove the effectiveness of both new and old drugs. This has led first to increasing sample size and increasing site numbers to overpower dwindling drug placebo differences, then to transferring studies out of the US to the third world, and now to quitting the field by many in Pharma. Simultaneously our discipline is criticized for manufacturing psychiatric disorders for the sake of corporate profit, and hoodwinking everyone into thinking that our drugs work whereas these are really dangerous chemicals that do harm and are no more effective than placebo for corporate disease-mongering of illnesses that do not exist to be treated by drugs that do not work to the mutual enrichment of Pharma and their investigators. Thus, this might also be our age of foolishness, our epoch of incredulity, our season of darkness, and our winter of despair.

What went wrong? In part, this book is an answer to that question and a proposal for the way forward. As explained in the chapters here by the world's leading experts, the solution is to combine the best methodologies, investigators, monitors, and, yes, new chemical entities. It requires understanding the science, the regulations, and the commercial imperatives of how this game of clinical trials is played and played to win.

We start with a background on the history of CNS drug development, and then an overview of regulatory issues, followed by a step-by-step progression through the clinical development process, from preclinical through approval. A unique aspect of our journey through CNS drug development is discussions of clinical trials management.

Although it is true that our discipline has a "worst of times" set of problems, we hope to show the way forward to deliver on the promise of new therapeutic agents for the CNS.

Stephen M. Stahl

History of CNS drug development

Sheldon Preskorn

Introduction

The intent of this chapter is to provide a conceptual framework for the rest of the book from both a historical and a forward-looking perspective.

Like all of medicine, drug development in psychiatry began with a series of chance discoveries from the 1930s to the 1960s. These drugs in large measure validated the following psychiatric syndromes: manic-depressive illness or bipolar (affective) disorder (i.e., lithium), unipolar affective disorder or major depression (i.e., iproniazid and imipramine), schizophrenia (i.e., chlorpromazine), and anxiety disorder (i.e., barbiturates, then meprobamate, and subsequently diazepam). Those initial drugs began the re-medicalization of psychiatry and served as probes into brain function which provided a means of better understanding the mechanisms underlying their clinical effects and thus the potential pathophysiology underlying these psychiatric syndromes (Goodwin and Preskorn, 1982; Preskorn, 1990).

Those drugs also permitted the development of technology (e.g., specific receptor binding) that permitted the rational development of newer drugs starting in the late 1960s and early 1970s and continuing to the current day. However, the rational development of psychiatric drugs in the 1970s and 1980s was generally limited to improving upon the pharmacology of the chance discovery drugs rather than developing truly novel medications. That was due to the limited understanding of the biology under both psychiatric and neurological diseases.

From the period of the 1980s to the current day, three other and inter-related developments occurred: (a) the industrialization of drug development process, (b) the dependency of major pharmaceutical companies ("big pharma") on the "blockbuster" (i.e., drugs that could generate one billion or more dollars in revenue per year) business model, and (c) the adoption of a commodity (e.g., soap) style marketing and sales approach (e.g., "new and improved Tide"). Until recently, block busters have generally been drugs which treated large percentages of the population (i.e., common diseases) chronically. That in turn means that the drug must be safe, well tolerated and effective for a large number of people and not just in one country but throughout the world, which in turn means not being susceptible to adverse interactions with the increased biological variance inherent in the world population.

The dependency on blockbuster drugs in turn has led to the industrialization of the drug development process and an emphasis on speed (to save patent life and thus maximize potential revenue, i.e., a month delay could translate into a loss of $100 million in

Essential CNS Drug Development, ed. A. Kalali, Sheldon Preskorn, J. Kwentus, and Stephen M. Stahl. Published by Cambridge University Press. © Cambridge University Press 2012.

revenue for a drug capable of generating $1.2 billion a year revenue). Following the adage that haste makes waste, the urgency to shorten the drug development process has set the stage for both the increase in the placebo response and the increased failure rate of drug development programs.

CNS drug development is at a critical fork in the road: (a) the promise of an increased ability to develop truly novel drugs and to better target those drugs for specific subsets of the populations and (b) the implosion of the blockbuster business model. The latter has led to the recent decision by two major pharmaceutical companies to stop developing drugs for psychiatric indications.

This chapter will cover these big picture topics by principally focusing on drug development for psychiatric as opposed to other central nervous system (CNS) indications such as neurological conditions, pain, and sleep. That decision was made to keep the chapter within the length guidelines established for it. Nevertheless, the principles outlined in this chapter are generally applicable to the development of drugs for these other indications. In addition, specific comments will be made about drugs for senile dementia of the Alzheimer's type, which, like a number of other neuropsychiatric conditions, falls outside the division between psychiatry and neurology.

Early drugs

Before discussing specific new early CNS drugs, the following is important from a historical perspective: the modern era of clinical psychopharmacology owes its beginnings to antibiotics, beginning with Fleming's discovery of penicillin in the 1920s and further enhanced by World War II (Geddes, 2008; Demain and Sanchez, 2009; Ligon, 2004). Fleming accidentally dropped crumbs of moldy bread into Petri dishes in which he was growing bacteria over a weekend. When he returned, he found that bacterial growth had been prevented in the areas of the Petri dishes where the bread crumbs had fallen. He concluded that there must be an antibacterial factor in the mold. He therefore set out to isolate that factor, which he subsequently called penicillin. World War II provided the incentive and the financial backing to develop methods for mass production of penicillin to treat infections secondary to combat trauma (Keefer, 1970; Richards, 1964). That was the basis for launching the pharmaceutical industry that exists today.

The contribution of antibiotic pharmacology to modern clinical pharmacology goes further: once an effective antibiotic was isolated from a plant (i.e., mold), organic (or medicinal) chemists could begin modifying the structure to develop new variations which (a) were patentable, (b) were capable of being reliably synthesized in commercial quantities, and (c) had some demonstrable and hence commercial advantage such as improved efficacy, safety, tolerability, or ease of administration when compared to an older antibiotic. This same approach became the universal approach in all therapeutic areas including CNS medications.

Table 1 lists the first drugs in psychiatry and the decade they were initially discovered.

These early drugs were principally discovered in two ways. The first was by observing the medicinal effects of plants. That approach dates back to before written history. The second occurred with the evolution of organic chemistry, permitting first the isolation and characterization of the active ingredients in plants (e.g., penicillin) and followed by the

Table 1. The early CNS drugs, class, and decade of discovery for a CNS indication

Drug	Class	Decade of discovery
Amphetamine	stimulant	1880s AD (Google, 2010)
Cocaine	analgesic/stimulant	1830s AD (Google, 2010)
Chlorpromazine	antipsychotic	1950s AD (Lopez-Munoz *et al.*, 2005)
Diazepam	anti-anxiety	1950s AD (http://itech.dickinson.edu/chemistry/?p=497, 2008)
Imipramine	antidepressant	1950s AD (Maxwell and Eckhardt, 2009)
Isocarboxazid	antidepressant	1950s AD (Darling *et al.*, 1959)
Lithium	mood stabilizer	1940s AD (Prien *et al.*, 1971)
Morphine	analgesic	2100 BC (Norn *et al.*, 2005)
Phenobarbital	anticonvulsant	1930s AD (Brink, 2010)
Reserpine	antipsychotic	1950s AD (Stitzel, 1976; Preskorn, 2007)

synthesis of new molecular entities which could then be manufactured in large quantities. Morphine and reserpine are examples of the former while chlorpromazine and imipramine are examples of the latter.

From chance to science: from chlorpromazine to newer antipsychotics and antidepressants

Chlorpromazine was a discovery which had its origins in the German aniline dye industry of the late 1800s and early 1990s (Lopez-Munoz *et al.*, 2005). Chlorpromazine and other phenothiazine molecules were synthesized around the turn of the last century and some were initially used to treat pinworm infestation. However, chlorpromazine over the last 50 years has come to play a pivotal role in the modern era of clinical psychopharmacology. This modern era began in large measure with Henri-Marie Laborit, M.D., a French surgeon, who recognized the calming effects that chlorpromazine exerted in anxious French patients going to surgery. Based on that observation, Dr. Laborit encouraged his French psychiatric colleagues to use it in French patients with anxiety disorders. They in turn found that chlorpromazine did have anti-anxiety effects at low dose (i.e., what they termed minor tranquilizing effects) and so they also tried it in agitated psychotic individuals. To their amazement, chlorpromazine at higher dose not only calmed agitated psychotic patients but actually reduced their psychotic symptoms (i.e., what they termed major tranquilizing effects). That observation ushered in the modern era of antipsychotic medications.

Soon after this discovery, chemists began working to tweak the phenothiazine structure of chlorpromazine to produce new drugs. Through such work, they produced other "low potency" antipsychotics such as thioridazine and clozapine (synthesized in 1960) and high potency phenothiazines such as trifluoroperazine and fluphenazine. They also produced derivatives which were, to their chagrin, inactive as antipsychotics

Chlorpromazine

low potency phenothiazine	high potency phenothiazine	imipramine and other TCAs
↓	↓	↓
clozapine	haloperidol	newer antidepressants (Figure 2)
↓	↓	
newer atypical antipsychotics	aripiprazole	

Figure 1. From chlorpromazine to conventional and atypical antipsychotics and TCAs.

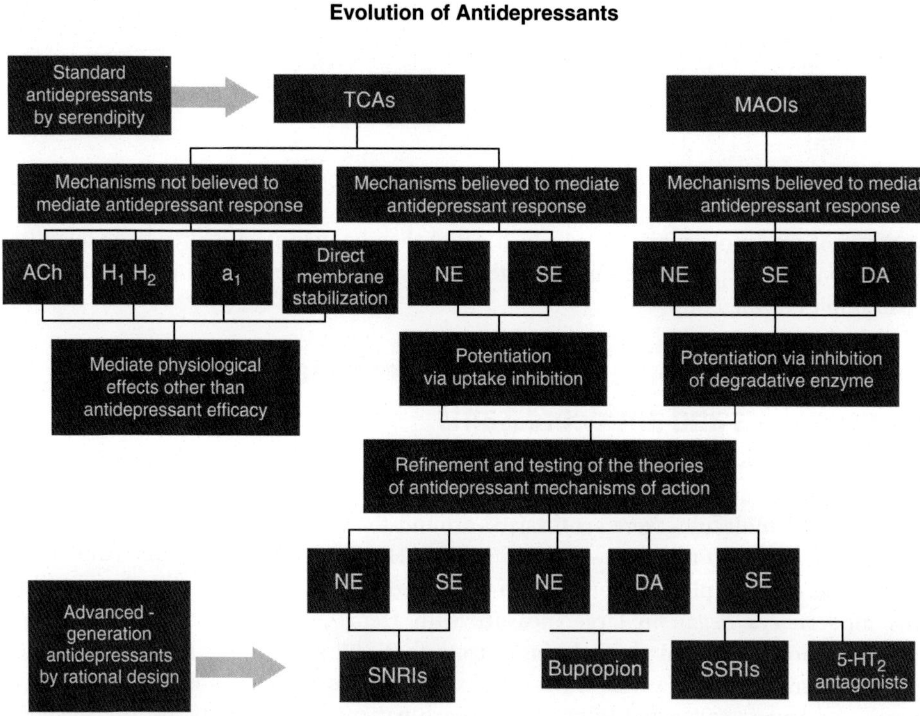

Evolution of Antidepressants

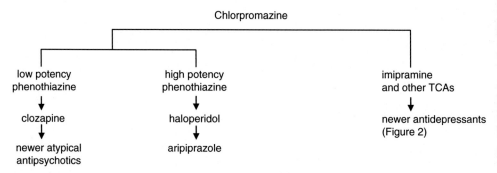

Figure 2. From TCAs and MAOIs to newer antidepressants. See plate section for color version.

but to their surprise, active as antidepressants (e.g., imipramine). Thus, chlorpromazine gave birth to atypical and conventional antipsychotics and to tricyclic antidepressants (TCAs) (Figure 1). As discussed below, TCAs together with monoamine oxidase inhibitors gave birth to all of the other newer antidepressants we have today including serotonin selective reuptake inhibitors (SSRIs) and serotonin-norepinephrine reuptake inhibitors (SNRIs) (Figure 2) (Lopez-Munoz and Alamo, 2009; Moncrieff, 2008; Preskorn, 1996).

Parenthetically, due to commodity marketing and sales, psychiatrists now widely believe that there are two generations of antipsychotic medications: conventional and atypical (Weiden *et al.*, 2007). They further believe that atypical antipsychotics are a new development. In fact, chlorpromazine – the first generally successful antipsychotic – and most of the other low potency phenothiazines meet most of the criteria as atypical antipsychotics (Preskorn, 2001) (Table 1). So "atypicality" is not new but old. The advertisements for thioridazine in the 1960s and 1970s are hardly distinguishable from the advertisements for newer antipsychotics. In fact, the advertising "war" in that era was between thioridazine and haloperidol, which was the new drug on the block touting its selective effects only on dopamine (D)-2 receptors without all of the other effects of thioridazine. Thus, there are actually four generations of antipsychotics: (a) the early atypicals such as chlorpromazine, thioridazine, and clozapine, (b) the selective D-2 pure antagonists (e.g., haloperidol), (c) the newer atypicals, and (d) the partial D-2 agonist (e.g., aripiprazole). What are now referred to as conventional antipsychotics means selective D-2 antagonists and does not properly include the low potency phenothiazines. The adjective "low potency" refers to the fact that these drugs have lower binding affinity for D-2 receptors than they do for other receptors. An unintended consequence of the commodity marketing seen as necessary to achieve blockbuster status is that the credibility of the pharmaceutical industry has fallen (i.e., commodity marketing and sales require that the drug must be new and improved even if the claims are only partially correct). That would have only affected physicians were it not for direct to consumer advertising, which has changed the image of big pharma from an enterprise aimed at improving the human condition to one akin to soap and automobile companies (i.e., selling product) (Huh *et al.*, 2010).

The era of the 1960s: understanding basic CNS pharmacology and developing early animal models of CNS diseases

The late 1950s and particularly the decade of the 1960s was a period of rapid growth in the understanding of biogenic amine (i.e., dopamine (D), norepinephrine (NE) and serotonin (5-HT)) transmitter systems in the brain, with Jules Alexrod and others leading the charge. During this period, the CNS anatomy of the biogenic amine neurotransmitter systems was mapped. The enzymatic pathways for their synthesis and degradation were elucidated as well as the mechanisms mediating their release, their reuptake and their pre- and post-synaptic receptors. That was accomplished in large part by studying the CNS pharmacology of the early CNS drugs (Table 1). Jules Axelrod received a Nobel Prize in 1970 for the work conducted in his lab on these issues (http://nobelprize.org/nobel_prizes/medicine/laureates/1970/axelrod-bio.html, 1972).

Scientists used the pharmacology of these early drugs to develop the initial theories of the pathophysiology of psychotic and depressive disorders (i.e., the hyper-dopamine theory of schizophrenia and the deficiency of biogenic amine theory of major depression) (Tost *et al.*, 2010). They also used the effects of these drugs to produce the first animal models of psychiatric illness, such as the dopamine hyperactivity model produced in a variety of ways such as intoxicating rats and other rodents with amphetamines to produce species-specific stereotypic movements. This was used to screen for D-2 selective antagonists such as haloperidol, which for 20 years during the decades of the 1970s and 1980s dominated the treatment of patients with schizophrenia and other psychotic disorders (Ayd, 1980; Demuth and Ackerman, 1983). In an analogous way, reserpine, tetrabenzapine

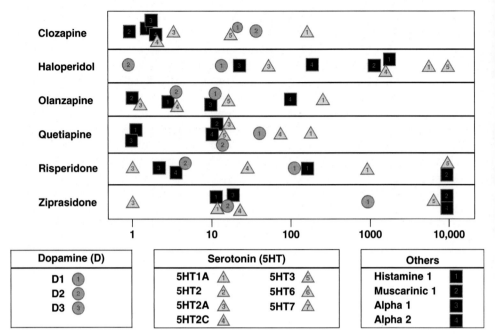

Figure 3. Comparison of the binding affinity of chlorpromazine, haloperidol and newer "atypical" antipsychotics. The profile for each drug is expressed relative to its most potent binding. See plate section for color version.

and various neurotoxic derivatives of amphetamine (e.g., para-chloramphetamine) were used to deplete the rodent brain of one or more of the biogenic amine neurotransmitters to serve as an animal model of depressive illness in humans.

Another important development in this period was the ability to isolate specific neurotransmitter receptors in test tubes by brain fractionation (Iversen et al., 1975). Via the development of this technology, scientists could begin to study the structure-activity relationship that allowed a drug to have high affinity for one receptor and low affinity for another. That work set the stage for the next era in the modern clinical psychopharmacology: the 1970s and 1980s.

The era of the 1970s and 1980s: redesigning drugs based on receptor pharmacology

Using receptor binding affinity, drug development scientists in the pharmaceutical industry produced new molecular entities using the theories and the techniques developed in the 1950s and 1960s. They either added binding affinities to specific proteins in the case of antipsychotic drugs or reduced them in the case of antidepressants to produce new molecules capable of being patented and simultaneously having truly desirable effects over existing drugs which could be touted by the marketing and sales departments of big pharma.

That was done by establishing the structure-activity relationship needed to mimic some but not all of the effects of the chance discovery drugs. In the case of the newer atypical antipsychotics, the goal was to produce molecules with higher binding affinity

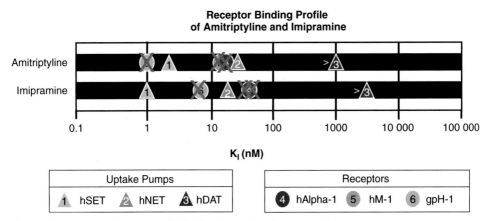

Figure 4. Receptor binding profile of TCAs. See plate section for color version.

for the 5-HT 2A receptor versus the D-2 receptor and minimally or no effects of early low potency phenothiazine on histamine-1 (H-1), muscarinic-1 acetylcholine (M-1), and alpha-1 norepinephrine (alpha-1) receptors (Preskorn, 2009b; Seeman, 2002) (Figure 3). The blockade of those three receptors caused the following generally unwanted effects: sedation and weight gain, peripheral and central anticholinergic effects, and orthostatic hypotension, respectively. In the case of antidepressants, the goal was also to simplify the pharmacology of the TCAs, principally by eliminating their effects on fast sodium channels which mediated their dose-dependent and serious cardiotoxicity and also eliminating their high binding affinity for the H-1, M-1, and alpha-1 receptors (Preskorn, 1996; Preskorn and Irwin, 1982) (Figure 4). As with the early low potency phenothiazines, blockade of those three receptors caused considerable tolerability problems for patients on TCAs. Given that they were analogs of low potency phenothiazines, TCAs not surprisingly shared some of the same pharmacology. In essence, the SSRIs and – even more so – the SNRIs were the TCAs without their limitations, as illustrated in Figure 5.

The major advance of the SSRIs and SNRIs was the fact that they were essentially not lethal when taken in an overdose whereas TCAs were for the prior 25 years the leading cause of death resulting from overdoses in many countries. The reason is that patients treated with antidepressants are prone to attempt suicide and one way is to take an overdose of your medications. Due to the narrow gap between their ability to inhibit the SE and NE uptake pumps versus the fast sodium channels, even a modest overdose of a TCA could be lethal.

While the tweaking of the receptor binding profile of the SSRIs, SNRIs, and the newer atypical antipsychotics did improve the tolerability and safety of these new medications compared to their forerunners, it did not change the mechanisms of action that mediated their desired clinical effects. That is consistent with the fact that the response and remission rates with the newer drugs are not better than those of the older medications and the substantial overlap in their efficacy, given that only a small portion of patients who do not respond to SSRIs will respond when switched to either SNRIs or TCAs (Preskorn, 2009a).

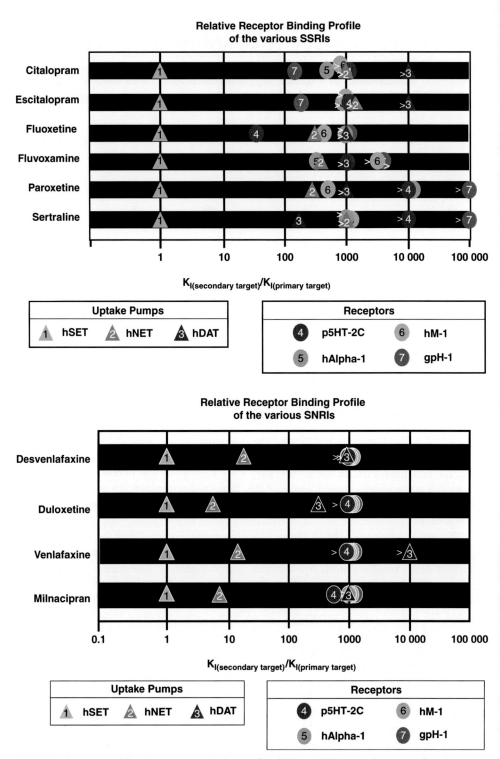

Figure 5. Comparison of the relative receptor binding profile of SSRIs and SNRIs. See plate section for color version.

The human genome project and its implications

The need now is to develop truly novel CNS drugs which work by new mechanisms of action. The hope here is with the human genome project and improved understanding of the molecular biology underlying psychiatric and neurological illnesses. The future can be seen in the dramatic advances being made in medicine for various forms of cancer (Kaelin, 1999; Lai, 2006).

However, there are multiple problems to be solved. The first is that the human genome project has a multitude of potential novel targets for drug development without enough information to know which ones are likely to be the most fruitful for drug development. It has been said that the major effect of the human genome project to date has been to increase the "burn rate" of pharmaceutical companies.

This problem is further amplified by the fact that the blockbuster model may no longer be viable (i.e., one drug to treat a large segment of the population) (Gilbert *et al.*, 2003; www.egonzehnder.com/global/download/issue1bigpharma.pdf, 2008). The reason is that improved knowledge of the molecular biology underlying psychiatric and neurological illnesses may result in splintering what appear now to be one common syndromic illness (e.g., major depression) into multiple better defined illnesses when understood from the level of pathophysiology or pathoetiology. That outcome has occurred in oncology but the approach has been to simply charge more money for the newer drugs to recoup the investment in drug development and turn a profit for the shareholder. The question is whether the same recoup of investment can be made in the case of psychiatric and neurological illnesses given that patients with these illnesses often cannot effectively advocate for themselves and have to rely on others to do that for them.

Two additional contributors to the current dilemma in drug development for psychiatric and neurological conditions are: (a) the cost of drug development due to regulatory hurdles and (b) the industrialization of the drug development process which has occurred over the last 20 years partially in response to the aforementioned cost. The Western world, particularly perhaps the USA, is risk averse. Hence, regulatory agencies (e.g., the Food and Drug Administration in the USA) have been established to protect society from having unsafe drugs on the market. The problem is that medicines with powerful effects on illnesses are likely to produce adverse effects in some individuals as a result of the same mechanisms that produce benefit. That problem is further aggravated by not knowing which people may be at risk for such adverse effects because of either genetic variations, concomitant diseases, or being on other medications. The other problem is that errors of commission (i.e., approving a drug later found to be unsafe in some patients) are more easily detected and likely to be punished than are errors of omission (i.e., discouraging the development of new drugs for serious conditions by making development too costly and too speculative). That can be seen today in the lack of the development of new antibiotics and we are likely seeing the same phenomenon in the decision by companies such as AstraZeneca and GlaxoSmithKline to abandon the development of new psychiatric medications.

The higher hurdle posed by increased expectations for drug development (i.e., number of patients tested and the types of studies done (e.g., thorough QTc studies)) creates two inter-related problems: (a) the process costs more in terms of both money and time and (b) the longer time-line leads to less time left to obtain a return on investment if the drug gets approved.

Industrialization of clinical trials was one solution that pharma developed to address the time-line problem. However, it has now become part of the problem. In this case industrialization refers to several common components of the current drug development process as follows: rigid time-lines for moving drugs from preclinical pharmacology to Phase I and then into Phase II and III; extensive boiler plate inclusion and exclusion criteria which severely limit the number of patients who can enter clinical trials; and the development of clinical trial sites as specialized, for-profit service providers to industry. This approach developed in the 1980s and 1990s when industry was developing drugs which were refinements of already existing drugs (as discussed above) rather than novel drugs with novel mechanisms of action. While there were good reasons for this industrialization in that era, this approach may not work well in the new era when there is greater uncertainty about what to pursue and how to do it.

During the 1980s and 1990s and into the early 2000s, CNS drug development was principally focused on SSRIs, SNRIs, "atypical" antipsychotics, and cholinesterase inhibitors. The SSRIs and SNRIs were derivates of tricyclic antidepressants. The "atypical" antipsychotics were derivates of clozapine. The cholinesterase inhibitors pursued the pathway blazed by tacrine. The endpoints and the time course for the trials were based on what was known from their predecessors. The question now is whether the paradigms and constructs established for drugs which principally affect different forms of biogenic amine neurotransmission are applicable to drugs that may work in fundamentally different ways.

As more about the biology of psychiatric illnesses becomes known, there may be a profound change in the way psychiatric illnesses are understood and codified. Current syndromes may be merged and subdivided in ways distinctly different from the current nomenclature. Treatments may be focused less on symptomatic relief and more on prevention. Such developments would make the current way of developing CNS drugs as antiquated as the buggy whip with the emergence of the gasoline engine.

This book then may be at the beginning of an era when the way CNS drugs are developed may need to be re-thought. If so, that will require flexibility and inherently involves uncertainty, which in turn means risk.

Development of drugs for Alzheimer's disease: a possible model for the future

The current development of drugs for Alzheimer's and other neurodegenerative diseases could be a model for how future CNS drug development might proceed (Becker and Greig, 2008; Bradford, 2002; Chico et al., 2009; Cummings, 2008; Markou et al., 2009; Pritchard, 2008; Steinmetz and Spack, 2009). The current treatments (e.g., donepezil) are symptomatic only and do not alter the course of the illness.

However, several theories about the underlying pathogenesis of Alzheimer's disease have been developed. These theories are based on histopathology, biochemistry, and molecular biology. Over 100 years ago, the microscopic pathology of the illness was known: amyloid plaques, neurofibrillary tangles, and the atrophy and eventual death of neurons. These lesions have now been subjected to biochemical analysis to identify their constituent parts (e.g., beta amyloid 1–42).

From a molecular biology standpoint, there are autosomal dominant forms of Alzheimer's disease. While these cases account for only approximately 1% of Alzheimer's cases, understanding the genetic basis of these cases has the potential to shed light on the biology of the more sporadic cases of Alzheimer's disease. The latter may be due to less severe defects in the same genes and may hence require multiple smaller genetic effects with or without the interaction of such genes and environmental factors. A number of genes identified from the autosomal dominant forms of Alzheimer's disease code for proteins that are involved in either the production of the abnormal proteins found in neurofibrillary tangles and/or amyloid plaques or clearance of these abnormal proteins (e.g., apolipoprotein E4). Based on these findings, theories about the biochemical pathogenesis of Alzheimer's disease have been developed. These theories in turn have spurred drug discovery aimed at intervening at the various steps in the proposed pathogenesis of the human disease, and are principally aimed at either decreasing the production of abnormal proteins and/or increasing their clearance.

Moreover, the transfer of the identified defective human genes into rodent embryos has produced adult animals which display to varying degrees the histopathology and functional impairment seen in human Alzheimer's disease. The hope and goal are to produce animal models which actually share the pathophysiology and pathogenesis underlying the human illness in contrast to the Porsolt learned helplessness model for depressive illnesses or various dopamine hyperactivity rodent models for schizophrenia. The new transgenic models have the potential to allow for testing of mechanism-based alteration in the biology of the illness.

This mechanism-based drug development has now been extended to individuals with Alzheimer's disease with the early endpoints being to determine whether the treatment produces a reduction in the concentration of the abnormal proteins either by decreasing their production and/or increasing their clearance. Those concentrations have been measured in both plasma and cerebrospinal fluid. Additional endpoints are to measure stopping loss of brain volume either generally or in specific areas such as hippocampal volume and also to quantitate the reduction in amyloid plaque density in the brain. Conceivably, such drugs might initially be approved for such endpoints rather than for changing the course of the illness in terms of memory or other functional impairment, much like the statin drugs were initially approved for their ability to lower lipids rather than to prevent atherosclerosis.

This new approach to drug development for Alzheimer's disease is in stark contrast to that for the development of the cholinesterase inhibitors, which were based on symptomatic maintenance of cognitive functioning. If successful, the application of this type of new treatment would ideally be for individuals at risk of developing Alzheimer's disease rather than for individuals who are already substantially impaired by the illness. The development of such treatment thus requires a substantial change in the paradigm of drug development for this therapeutic area in terms of study design and site capabilities. It is also hypothesis-driven in a much more refined and technologically advanced way with "harder" (i.e., more quantifiable) endpoints compared to "softer" symptomatic rating scale endpoints. While this area is exciting, it remains to be seen whether it will result in the approval of truly game-changing medications. The history of medicine and science suggests that it will. Hence, the more apt question is: when?

The next question is: when will enough be known about the pathophysiology and pathogenesis of other brain diseases such as schizophrenia, bipolar disorder, and major depression to pursue this same approach for the development of new treatments for these illnesses? That raises the further question: how different will the development of such drugs be from what has been the case to date for antipsychotics, mood stabilizers, and antidepressants? How much will such treatments change the nature of when these illnesses are treated and their impact on the lives of those who have suffered from them and their families and society in general?

This chapter then has endeavored to provide an overview of how CNS drug development has evolved over its relatively short history of perhaps 50–100 years as well as to provide some sense of how it might evolve in the not-too-distant future. The rest of the book will provide more depth into each of the steps and facets of this process and journey.

References

Ayd, J. F. (Ed.) (1980). *Haloperidol Update: 1958–1980*. Baltimore: Ayd Medical Communications.

Becker, R. E. and Greig, N. H. (2008). Alzheimer's disease drug development in 2008 and beyond: problems and opportunities. *Curr Alzheimer Res*, 5, 346–57.

Bradford, L. D. (2002). CYP2D6 allele frequency in European Caucasians, Asians, Africans and their descendants. *Pharmacogenomics*, 3, 229–43.

Brink, C. J. (2010). [Phenobarbital]. *Tijdschr Diergeneeskd*, 135, 248; author reply 248–9.

Chico, L. K., Van Eldik, L. J., and Watterson, D. M. (2009). Targeting protein kinases in central nervous system disorders. *Nat Rev Drug Discov*, 8, 892–909.

Cummings, J. L. (2008). Controversies in Alzheimer's disease drug development. *Int Rev Psychiatry*, 20, 389–95.

Darling, H. F., Kruse, W., Hess, G. F., and Hoermann, M. G. (1959). Preliminary study of isocarboxazid, an iproniazid analog. *Dis Nerv Syst*, 20, 269–71.

Demain, A. L. and Sanchez, S. (2009). Microbial drug discovery: 80 years of progress. *J Antibiot (Tokyo)*, 62, 5–16.

Demuth, G. W. and Ackerman, S. H. (1983). alpha-Methyldopa and depression: a clinical study and review of the literature. *Am J Psychiat*, 140, 534–8.

Geddes, A. (2008). 80th Anniversary of the discovery of penicillin. An appreciation of Sir Alexander Fleming. *Int J Antimicrob Agents*, 32, 373.

Gilbert, J., Henske, P., and Singh, A. (2003). Rebuilding Big Pharma's Business Model. *IN VIVO The Business & Medicine Report*. Winhover Information Inc.

Goodwin, D. W. and Preskorn, S. H. (1982). DSM-III and pharmacotherapy. In Turner, S. and Hersen, M. (Eds.), *Adult Psychopathology: A Social Work Perspective*. New York: John Wiley and Sons.

Google (2010). Early history of amphetamine – Google Search. Google.

http://itech.dickinson.edu/chemistry/?p=497 (2008). History of Diazepam. The Role of Chemistry in History.

http://nobelprize.org/nobel_prizes/medicine/laureates/1970/axelrod-bio.html (1972). Julius Axelrod – Biography.

Huh, J., Delorme, D. E., Reid, L. N., and An, S. (2010). Direct-to-consumer prescription drug advertising: history, regulation, and issues. *Minn Med*, 93, 50–2.

Iversen, L. L., Iversen, S. D., and Snyder, S. H. (Eds.) (1975). *Handbook of Psychopharmacology*. New York: Plenum Press.

Kaelin, W. G., Jr. (1999). Choosing anticancer drug targets in the postgenomic era. *J Clin Invest*, 104, 1503–6.

Keefer, C. S. (1970). Alfred Newton Richards in Washington as Chairman of the World War 2 Committee on Medical Research, he brought penicillin from the test tube to full production. *Med Aff*, 32, 8–11 passim.

Lai, C. W. (2006). Pharmacogenomics: methods and protocols. *Brit J Cancer*, 94, 1553.

Ligon, B. L. (2004). Penicillin: its discovery and early development. *Semin Pediatr Infect Dis*, 15, 52–7.

Lopez-Munoz, F. and Alamo, C. (2009). Monoaminergic neurotransmission: the history of the discovery of antidepressants from 1950s until today. *Curr Pharm Des*, 15, 1563–86.

Lopez-Munoz, F., Alamo, C., Cuenca, E., Shen, W. W., Clervoy, P., and Rubio, G. (2005). History of the discovery and clinical introduction of chlorpromazine. *Ann Clin Psychiat*, 17, 113–35.

Markou, A., Chiamulera, C., Geyer, M. A., Tricklebank, M., and Steckler, T. (2009). Removing obstacles in neuroscience drug discovery: the future path for animal models. *Neuropsychopharmacology*, 34, 74–89.

Maxwell, R. A. and Eckhardt, S. B. (2009). *Drug Discovery: A Casebook and Analysis*. New York: Springer.

Moncrieff, J. (2008). The creation of the concept of an antidepressant: an historical analysis. *Soc Sci Med*, 66, 2346–55.

Norn, S., Kruse, P. R., and Kruse, E. (2005). [History of opium poppy and morphine]. *Dan Medicinhist Arbog*, 33, 171–84.

Preskorn, S. H. (1990). The future and psychopharmacology: potentials and needs. *Psychiat Ann*, 20, 625–33.

Preskorn, S. H. (1996). *Clinical Pharmacology of Selective Serotonin Reuptake*. Caddo, OK: Professional Communications Inc.

Preskorn, S. H. (2001). Antipsychotic drug development in the pre-human-genome era: a full circle. *J Psychiatr Pract*, 7, 209–13.

Preskorn, S. H. (2007). The evolution of antipsychotic drug therapy: reserpine, chlorpromazine, and haloperidol. *J Psychiatr Pract*, 13, 253–7.

Preskorn, S. H. (2009a). Results of the STAR*D study: implications for clinicians and drug developers. *J Psychiatr Pract*, 15, 45–9.

Preskorn, S. H. (2009b). A roadmap to key pharmacologic principles in using antipsychotics: application in clinical practice. *J Clin Psychiat*, 70, 593–600.

Preskorn, S. H. and Irwin, H. A. (1982). Toxicity of tricyclic antidepressants – kinetics, mechanism, intervention: a review. *J Clin Psychiat*, 43, 151–6.

Prien, R. F., Caffey, E. M., Jr., and Klett, C. J. (1971). Lithium carbonate. A survey of the history and current status of Lithium in treating mood disorders. *Dis Nerv Syst*, 32, 521–31.

Pritchard, J. F. (2008). Risk in CNS drug discovery: focus on treatment of Alzheimer's disease. *BMC Neurosci*, 9 Suppl 3, S1.

Richards, A. N. (1964). Production of penicillin in the United States (1941–1946). *Nature*, 201, 441–5.

Seeman, P. (2002). Atypical antipsychotics: mechanism of action. *Can J Psychiat*, 47, 27–38.

Steinmetz, K. L. and Spack, E. G. (2009). The basics of preclinical drug development for neurodegenerative disease indications. *BMC Neurol*, 9 Suppl 1, S2.

Stitzel, R. E. (1976). The biological fate of reserpine. *Pharmacol Rev*, 28, 179–208.

Tost, H., Alam, T., and Meyer-Lindenberg, A. (2010). Dopamine and psychosis: theory, pathomechanisms and intermediate phenotypes. *Neurosci Biobehav Rev*, 34, 689–700.

Weiden, P. J., Preskorn, S. H., Fahnestock, P. A., Carpenter, D., Ross, R., and Docherty, J. P. (2007). Translating the psychopharmacology of antipsychotics to individualized treatment for severe mental illness: a Roadmap. *J Clin Psychiat*, 68 Suppl 7, 1–48.

www.egonzehnder.com/global/download/issue1bigpharma.pdf (2008). Big Pharma's New Leadership Models: Making them work. Egon Zehnder International.

Regulatory issues

Gwen L. Zornberg

As gatekeeper to the United States drug market, the Food and Drug Administration (FDA) presides over approval for use of new pharmaceuticals contingent upon the review of safety, efficacy, and quality. In this chapter, to better understand how new psychotropic drugs are approved for clinical use, we need to appreciate the complex evolution and drivers of the nation's drug approval process. It is critical to understand that the drug regulation system is constantly evolving in an expanding legal framework involving numerous players. Labeling is emphasized because it is the chief vehicle used by the regulatory agency and the manufacturer to communicate risks and benefits of drugs to patients and the healthcare community.

Introduction to the US drug approval process

What makes a drug a drug? The answer is the "intended use" as defined by law. Drugs are small molecules that are defined as articles (other than food) recognized by the United States Pharmacopeia (USP), the National Formulary, or the Homeopathic Pharmacopeia, which are intended for use in the diagnosis, cure, mitigation, treatment, or prevention of disease in human beings. The intended use is determined from labeling and claims made in promotion by the manufacturer who develops the drug product and submits applications to the FDA for approval. Labeling describes what the prescriber should know for proper use of the drug. While a label is the printed or graphic matter upon the immediate drug container, the term "labeling" conveys all labels and any printed, written, or graphic matter accompanying a container or wrapper such as package inserts, brochures, detailing pieces, motion pictures, film strips, exhibits, literature, reprints, mailing pieces, and similar pieces for use by clinicians to supplement and explain the intended use. It is the job of the FDA to ensure that beneficial medical products are available and labeled with accurate prescribing information. While the FDA regulates other therapeutics such as biologics, over the counter drugs, and medical devices, this chapter will provide an overview of the FDA's regulation of prescription drug products.

Congress created the FDA to regulate drugs introduced into interstate commerce in the USA to ensure their safety, efficacy, and quality. Regulations are governmental orders that are predicated on the interpretation of laws that the agency has been charged with implementing. FDA regulations and other communications are listed in the *Federal Register*, which publishes notice of proposed new rules and regulations, as well as final rules, changes to existing rules, notices of availability of guidances, meetings, and comments on

Essential CNS Drug Development, ed. A. Kalali, Sheldon Preskorn, J. Kwentus, and Stephen M. Stahl. Published by Cambridge University Press. © Cambridge University Press 2012.

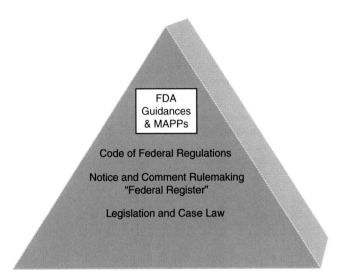

Figure 1. Statutory underpinnings of FDA Guidances.

rulemaking prior to finalization. Final rules published in the *Federal Register* are then codified into the Code of Federal Regulations. To convey the FDA's interpretation of or policy on a drug regulatory issue, the agency develops and issues guidance documents that are prepared for use by FDA staff, applicants/sponsors, and the public (Figure 1). Guidance documents include though are not limited to the processing, content, and evaluation or approval of submissions or the design, production, labeling, promotion, manufacturing, and testing of regulated products.

Numerous constituencies interact within the medical system where drugs are tested and used. Major players involved include manufacturers who develop drugs and submit the applications for review to the FDA; healthcare providers who prescribe, advise, and/or administer drug products; patients who require healthcare; and policy makers.

Applicable statutes

Regulation of pharmaceuticals in the United States began in 1906 with the federal Pure Food and Drugs Act that prohibited the sale of misbranded drugs or adulterated foods. Under the original Act, claims for drugs in labeling were permitted by default unless they were later proven by the agency to be inaccurate or misleading, i.e., misbranded. The mandate for truth in labeling put the burden of proof on the FDA.

The enactment of the Food, Drug, and Cosmetic Act (FD&C Act) of 1938 ushered in an era of greater emphasis on safety in pharmaceuticals. The FD&C Act, the principal source of authority for the FDA, provides the basic regulatory framework mandating that new drugs be shown to be safe by the manufacturer. The FD&C Act gives broad regulatory authority to the FDA to institute standards, approve new drug applications, ensure compliance, authorize factory inspections, and enforce the law. The FDA's authorities are largely devoted to pre-marketing and post-marketing risk-benefit evaluation. The Act was a regulatory game-changer by stipulating that the results of research must be submitted by manufacturers for approval in a New Drug Application (NDA) with labeling. This shifted the burden of proof from the FDA to the manufacturer.

Until the Durham-Humphrey Amendment of 1951, there was no law requiring that a drug should be labeled for sale only by prescription. Prescription drugs were defined as those unsafe for self-medication that should be used only under a physician's supervision.

In 1962, the Kefauver-Harris Drug Amendment ushered in an era of heightened focus on efficacy by requiring a positive act of approval by the FDA. New drugs must be demonstrated to be effective in applications – as well as safe. The NDA must contain "substantial evidence" of the drug's efficacy as well as safety for use in the targeted patient population. Moreover, the amendment required that the FDA reviewed all drugs that had entered the market since 1938. The Drug Efficacy Study Implementation (DESI) reviews were conducted by the National Academy of Sciences-National Research Council (NAS-NRC) beginning in 1966. The recommendations were published in the *Federal Register* as DESI notices. If found to be safe and effective, the drug remained on the market. If considered safe and probably effective, the drug remained on the market until finally approved based on sufficient data from additional efficacy studies. If evidence for safety and efficacy was absent, the drug was removed from the market.

With advancing science driving the development of burgeoning panoplies of new drugs, legislative consideration was made of certain intellectual property rights as part of the FDA's drug approval process. As a result, Congress enacted the 1984 Drug Price Competition and Patent Term Restoration Act (The "Waxman-Hatch Act") to resolve two competing goals. The growing demand for prompt and easier entry of generic drugs into competition on the market, which are usually sold at lower cost, was balanced with the need to encourage new drug innovation. To strengthen drug price competition through the development of generic drugs, this law expands the numbers of drugs suitable for use of the less cumbersome and less costly Abbreviated NDAs (ANDAs). To reward innovation, "Patent Term Restoration" refers to the 17 years of legal protection granted to the applicant for each drug patent. A certain proportion of the 17 year time allowance is spent while the drug goes through the approval process, so this law allows through the FDA approval process for restoration of up to 5 years of lost patent time.

To facilitate the introduction of innovative new drugs into clinical use, the 1992 Prescription Drug User Fee Act (PDUFA) and its reauthorizations introduced and then established user fees to provide the resources needed to achieve accelerated drug review goals. The objective of PDUFA is to allow earlier patient access to safe and effective new therapeutics without compromising standards. Implementation of PDUFA fees to optimize the efficiency of multidisciplinary reviews coupled with initiatives implemented by the Center for Drug Evaluation and Research (CDER) since the early 1990s have resulted in reduced NDA review times for new therapeutics (General Accounting Office report, FDA Drug Approval: Review Time has Decreased in Recent Years, http://www.fda.gov/AboutFDA/ReportsManualsForms/Reports/UserFeeReports/PerformanceReports/PDUFA/ucm117257.htm).

The FDA Modernization Act (FDAMA) of 1997 implemented considerable provisions expanding patient access to experimental drugs and medical devices, information on clinical trials, and other matters. FDAMA provided clarification of the concept of "substantial evidence" to support drug approval (*Guidance for Industry*, "Providing Clinical Evidence of Effectiveness for Human Drug and Biological Products", May, 1998). A provision allows manufacturers to disseminate peer-reviewed articles about unapproved uses of drugs provided that they commit to file within a specified timeframe to establish the safety and efficacy of the unapproved use for a period of five years. Due to growing public interest in innovative new drugs, FDAMA required the establishment of a clinical trial registry. This database, www.ClinicalTrials.gov, contains information on trials conducted in more than 160 countries.

As there had been few incentives to study drugs in children, the pediatric studies initiative was codified to fill the data gap on fundamental information on the product label for safe use of drugs in children and adolescents. To ensure compliance with pediatric research requirements, both "stick" and "carrot" strategies were employed. The "stick" approach was applied through the 1998 Final Pediatric Rule holding that pediatric studies are mandatory. In October 2002, the FDA was prohibited by a judicial order from enforcing the Pediatric Rule. The requirement for studies in pediatric populations became the law when codified under the 2003 Pediatric Research Equity Act (PREA). Consequently, if pediatric studies are deferred with NDA approval, the applicant must submit an annual review posted on the internet detailing progress made in conducting the deferred pediatric studies. In 2002, the Best Pharmaceuticals for Children Act (BPCA) reauthorized the "carrot" of pediatric exclusivity, i.e., equivalent to the extension of patent protection by 6 months for the study of drugs in children and adolescents. Pediatric exclusivity holds not just for the pediatric formulations or indications, but also for all protected indications and formulations of the drug product. If a waiver for the requirement to conduct pediatric studies is granted because there is evidence that the drug would likely be ineffective or unsafe, such information shall be included in labeling.

The impact of the Food and Drug Administration Amendments Act (FDAAA) of 2007 (Title IX) has been particularly far-reaching in shifting even greater emphasis on to new strategies to bolster drug safety. FDAAA provides new authorities to the FDA to require post-marketing safety studies and clinical trials as well as safety-related labeling changes. In certain circumstances of elevated safety risk, FDAAA mandates the development of a risk evaluation and mitigation strategy (REMS), a new type of risk management plan. Moreover, FDAAA increased the usefulness of the www.ClinicalTrials.gov database by requiring the availability through the website of more information related to clinical trials.

From drug discovery forward, disentangling spurious leads from the true profiles of new candidate drugs contributes to the resource-intensive nature of the development venture. Out of the growing framework of laws governing drug regulation, the FDA has established the gold standard for a well-defined pre-marketing review and approval process. The process draws on a series of post-marketing surveillance programs to gather data and assess risks as information accrues. The hope and expectation for each new drug will be a systematic and reasonably predictable review process from the initial application through to approval. Patients rely on this system to ensure that prescribed drugs are safe and effective for their intended medical uses.

The Investigational New Drug application (IND)

An investigational new drug is one that is used in a clinical investigation. The IND is unique to the regulatory process for drug approval in the United States. Clinical development of a new psychotropic drug, for example, begins when the sponsor submits an IND application to the FDA that generally includes data on a viable candidate in three broad areas:

- Animal pharmacology and toxicology studies
- Manufacturing information
- Clinical protocols and investigator information

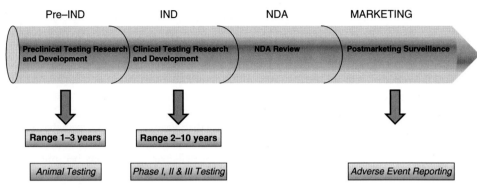

Figure 2. Drug development timeline.

The FDA has 30 days to review the IND to allow it to proceed or to impose a hold. A clinical hold is an order issued by the FDA to the sponsor to delay a proposed clinical investigation or to suspend an ongoing study. When a proposed study is placed on hold, participants may not be given the investigational drug by the clinical investigator conducting the study until the hold is lifted. The grounds for imposition of the hold of a study under an IND are that human subjects would be exposed to an unreasonable risk of harm; the clinical investigators are not qualified; the investigator brochure is misleading, erroneous, or materially incomplete; and/or the IND does not contain sufficient information to assess the risks to the study participants. Later in development, the finding that a study protocol is deficient in its design to meet its stated objectives may also be grounds to support a hold. Although the FDA provides advice on the development of experimental therapies allowed to proceed forward in clinical testing, investigators may choose to ignore advice regarding the design of studies in areas other than patient safety. Well-conducted IND research facilitates efficient drug development by ensuring patient safety, minimizing inaccurate or misleading results, and helping identify the optimal clinical dose-response range for the drug in the target patient population.

The FDA provides guidance on nonclinical testing requirements, i.e., animal testing preceding exposure in humans, particularly those pertaining to pharmacology and toxicology studies. The FDA requires preclinical in vitro and in vivo animal testing to evaluate the toxic and pharmacologic effects. Studies of acute toxicity of the drug must be conducted in at least two mammalian species, then short-term toxicity from 2 weeks to 3 months is evaluated. The acute toxicity studies should include dosages that are intended to cause no adverse effects and, at the other extreme, those intended to cause life-threatening toxicity. The research findings are extrapolated from animals to humans, aiming to reduce the risk and severity of drug-related toxicities. In order to assure the integrity of the safety data, Good Laboratory Practice (GLP) regulations are implemented to support marketing applications. GLP provides for comprehensive physical inspections of laboratory facilities and operations, in addition to data audits of laboratories that conduct animal safety testing of FDA-regulated products.

There are four phases that span the clinical drug development process, i.e., Phase I through Phase IV (Figure 2). The distinctions between the phases of clinical drug development are largely arbitrary. In Phase I, the primary question to be answered is whether the drug is safe in humans. Phase I studies are dose-finding studies designed to evaluate tolerability, safety, and pharmacokinetic and pharmacodynamic (PK/PD) parameters, as well as bioassay and drug-drug interactions. The IND must be submitted to the FDA before human testing is initiated once the applicant determines that sufficient nonclinical data have been garnered to support the expectation of a satisfactory safety profile and to determine a reasonable starting dose in humans. First-in-human single dose studies are followed by multiple escalating dose studies. The size of these closely monitored, controlled studies tends to be relatively small. Generally, only 20 to 80 healthy volunteers are enrolled. The FDA encourages full exploration of all doses within the therapeutic dose range and a full range of sampling times after dosing in order to fully characterize the pharmacokinetics of the drug.

In Phase II, the major clinical issue to be addressed becomes whether there is preliminary evidence of efficacy. Hence "proof of concept" type studies are undertaken to estimate the potential efficacy of the new drug for the intended use in patients. Adverse drug experiences are studied often at fixed doses. Drug formulation decisions are made at this stage as well as in Phase I. As preliminary confirmation of efficacy emerges, the sizes of the study populations tend to enlarge to several hundred participants for dose verification and evaluation of dose-response relationships. These data aid in refining criteria to identify the patient population and other aspects of study design in large Phase III multicenter, randomized, double-blind trials comparing the new psychotropic drug to treatment with placebo and possibly also to standard therapy.

In Phase III, the cardinal question now crystallizes into: "How safe and effective is the new drug for the intended use compared to other treatments?" Expanded Phase III confirmatory clinical trials represent the most definitive testing for unapproved drugs. Such "adequate and well-controlled" investigations are required to meet the evidentiary standard for approval. Generally, several hundred to a few thousand trial participants are studied in trials conducted over 2 to 3 years. Randomization is critical for confirmatory testing in the effort to achieve equipoise with a reduced likelihood of imbalances of prognostic factors such as age, sex, and comorbidity. Imbalances bias the analyses by distorting the estimates of treatment changes in the drug group compared to the control group. The study protocols to address the regulatory questions of interest must be reviewed under the IND by the FDA before the start of the trial. Key aspects of trial design required in the protocol include: objectives of the trial, qualifications of each investigator, patient selection criteria, study design, type of control group(s), clinical procedures, primary (and possibly key secondary) efficacy assessments, laboratory tests, and other measures to monitor safety effects of the drug while minimizing risk to trial participants. It is critical that the primary clinical endpoint assessment is specific for the condition under investigation.

The investigator obligations are to conduct the trial according to the protocol while protecting participant welfare. Any changes to the final study protocol must be submitted to the FDA as a protocol amendment. Documentation such as reports on progress, safety, and financial disclosure must be submitted and drug accountability must be maintained. As essential study documentation, information on the drug's adverse experience profile, pharmacology, and toxicology in the investigator brochure is updated annually (or sooner) through amendments. Case report forms are used to record data on all trial participants. Safety data from the trials are analyzed in the effort to elucidate the basis for observed or reported adverse drug experiences (ADEs). All of this is undertaken in keeping with Good Clinical Practice, which ensures that the study is well designed and follows scientific principles, that the IRB protects the safety and rights of participants including that informed consent is given freely, and that the data must be accurate and complete with quality assurance plans in place.

Expanded access to treatment

The main route of access to investigational drugs is through enrollment in a clinical trial. The FDA, however, has had a long-standing policy of facilitating access to investigational therapies for serious or life-threatening illnesses through informal mechanisms based on the agency's "reasonableness decision".

The FDA issued two new final rules in 2009 on expanded access to promising investigational drugs for treatment use. The first rule elucidates existing regulations and adds new types of expanded access for treatment use including availability for individual patients (e.g., for emergency use), in intermediate-size populations, as well as for larger populations under a treatment protocol (T-IND). Treatment INDs are employed for widespread treatment use when the drug is still in clinical trials or when the trials have been completed though the application has not yet been approved. There must be sufficient clinical evidence to support the expanded use for an individual. The second final rule amends the IND regulation on charging patients for investigational drugs. This rule elucidates when charging is permissible for an investigational drug in a clinical trial, it provides criteria for the different types of expanded access for treatment use, and it clarifies what costs can be recovered by the sponsor.

The New Drug Application (NDA)

Preparation of the NDA for successful submission necessitates ongoing communication between the FDA and the applicant to understand what is required for approval with a reasonable degree of predictability. There are a variety of informal and formal interactions between the applicant and the FDA on scientific, medical, and procedural issues. For instance, there are written communications such as information request letters from the agency to the applicant. Formal interactions between the FDA and the applicant also involve a variety of meetings such as end-of-Phase II conferences and pre-NDA meetings.

Standard NDAs have 10 month review times, though the review may take longer. Priority NDAs are allotted 6 month goal review times. Priority review may be granted if the drug would offer a significant improvement in filling an unmet therapeutic need for a serious or life-threatening condition (e.g., increased effectiveness, or elimination or substantial reduction of drug reaction over marketed products/therapies in the treatment, diagnosis, or prevention of disease).

CDER classifies NDAs with a code that reflects both the type of drug being submitted as well as the intended use(s). A "new molecular entity" (NME) is an active moiety that has not been previously approved or legally marketed as the active moiety in the United States in any drug product, either as the single ingredient, as part of a combination product, or as part of a mixture of stereoisomers. The drug classification system is determined by policy, not regulation or statute. The numbers one through eight are used for drug classification coding to describe the type of drug:

1. New molecular entity
2. New active ingredient (e.g., new salt of a previously approved drug) not an NME
3. New formulation of a previously approved drug (not a new salt or an NME)

4. New combination of two or more drugs
5. New manufacturer or new formulation (already marketed drug product)
6. New indication for an already marketed drug, same manufacturer
7. Already legally marketed drug – without approved NDA
8. Prescription to over the counter switch in marketing status

Once submitted, the NDA is forwarded to the appropriate CDER review division with required patent information and draft labeling. Within the first 60 days after receipt, the assigned cross-disciplinary NDA review team evaluates whether the application meets the minimum submission standards to be considered "fileable". The decision is communicated to the sponsor. Were the application to be considered incomplete (such as consisting of data not found to be usable), the FDA would issue a "refuse to file" letter.

The FDA has been streamlining and standardizing the process to facilitate more efficient reviews. This has been a daunting challenge for all involved. To begin with, the length of the average NDA is 100 000 pages or longer. Nonetheless, given the recognized efficiencies of standardized, consistent data formats to facilitate improved regulatory reviews, the FDA now requires the NDA to be submitted in an internationally harmonized, electronic "Common Technical Document" (eCTD) format. The new format reduces the time and resources required for NDA submission and review. The five modules of the eCTD format highlight the domains of in-depth data analyses to support the corresponding information in labeling. The modules are titled: Module 1, Administrative information and prescribing information in labeling; Module 2, Summaries and overview; Module 3, Information on product quality; Module 4, Nonclinical study toxicology and pharmacology reports; and Module 5, Clinical study reports. The integrated summary of effectiveness (ISE) and integrated summary of safety (ISS) of Module 5 of the eCTD contain the full reports of studies of efficacy and safety that are features unique to the NDA. Note that the terms ISE and ISS have caused confusion for sponsors regarding the required format for submissions in the CTD format. The term "Integrated Summary" suggests to some applicants that a brief overview would be expected. The succinct overviews, however, are found in Module 2 of the eCTD. In contrast, the ISE and ISS are detailed, integrated in-depth analyses of all clinical data pertaining to the efficacy and safety of the drug for the indication under review from the clinical trial study reports.

The components of the NDA tend to be relatively uniform. The quality and data, however, vary as they are in part a function of the drug under review and the information available to the applicant. As outlined in application Form FDA-356h, "Application to Market a New Drug, Biologic or an Antibiotic Drug for Human Use", NDAs can consist of as many as 15 different sections:

- Index
- Labeling
- Summary
- Chemistry (including quality, manufacturing, and controls; samples; and methods validation)
- Nonclinical pharmacology and toxicology
- Human pharmacokinetics and bioavailability
- Clinical microbiology (for anti-microbial drugs only)
- Clinical data

- Safety update report
- Statistical section
- Case-report tabulations
- Case-report forms
- Patent information
- Patent certification
- Other information

Based on the content of the electronically filed "eNDA", the appropriate divisions review the data in pertinent sections and draw on consultative reviews as necessary. Under consideration may be issues such as a drug's abuse potential, evaluation of exploratory pharmacogenetics data that may have been submitted, or consumer information detailed in labeling. The FD&C Act establishes that the sponsor must demonstrate that the new drug is:

- safe for use under the conditions prescribed in the labeling;
- effective for use under the conditions prescribed in the labeling based on substantial evidence from adequate and well-controlled investigations;
- produced with methods using chemistry, manufacturing, and controls that are adequate to preserve the identity, strength, quality, and purity of the drug.

Hence, the quality or chemistry, manufacturing, and controls section of the NDA contains complete lists of components, composition, the full description of manufacturing and controls, in addition to specifications of both the active ingredient and the drug product. The stability and physical and chemical characteristics of the drug product are provided for evaluation. The nonclinical section should provide all animal and laboratory data, including findings from the preclinical studies originally submitted in the IND up to submission of the NDA. This section of the NDA will include also long-term carcinogenicity studies and reproductive testing in animal models.

The clinical pharmacology reviewer evaluates data on the human pharmacokinetic and bioavailability studies, including a description of the analytical and statistical methods employed. The effect of factors such as age, body weight, and gender on pharmacokinetic parameters such as apparent volume of distribution and half-life are assessed. To the extent possible, the robustness of the pharmacokinetic and pharmacodynamic data is evaluated with respect to extrapolations to clinical efficacy and safety findings.

Efficacy evaluation

As a basis for approval, the FDA must ascertain whether the body of data in the application meets the evidentiary standard of adequate and well-controlled investigations that are convincing to experts qualified by scientific training and experience. Large, multicenter, placebo-controlled, randomized, double-blind trials of new psychotropic drugs are still considered the regulatory "gold standard" as confirmatory of safety and efficacy.

Often, the sponsor studies treatment groups of only one dose or possibly up to a few doses of the new drug in confirmatory trials. This strategy has the disadvantage of limiting the ability to evaluate for a dose-response effect on the clinical endpoint. The use of placebo control groups for psychiatric drug trials submitted to the FDA remains the standard for purposes of approval. This is largely because the effect estimates of psychotropic drugs often appear less robust than true drug effects due to the etiological and symptomatic heterogeneity of the patient populations, which tends to obscure the ability to detect mean group differences. Hence, a comparison between the new drug and an active control without a placebo group is only convincing when the new psychotropic is superior to the standard remedy. If the new drug is inferior to the active control, or even indistinguishable, the results are not readily interpretable without a concurrent placebo control. Were the new drug found to not be statistically superior to placebo, it would be considered a negative trial for regulatory purposes. In general, a positive controlled clinical trial with statistically significant results must be replicated for approval.

No psychiatric diagnostic subgroup has been consistently and validly identified by a biomarker or been genetically defined. FDA finds the identification of a diagnostic subpopulation acceptable for support of a labeling claim of an intended use if the clinical subgroup can be validly and reliably identified. For regulatory purposes, a diagnostic subgroup with a worse prognosis (e.g., treatment-resistant depression) will have a lower evidentiary bar than a subgroup with a theoretically better prognosis. The onus, however, remains on the applicant to demonstrate that the subpopulation is a real clinical entity.

CDER's "Critical Path Initiative" has heralded the FDA's concerted focus on targeted scientific efforts to modernize the techniques and methods used to evaluate the safety, efficacy, and quality of drugs from product selection to manufacturing. FDA is addressing the limitations of traditional clinical trial designs with fixed sample sizes and other conventional design features to allow more flexible, efficient approaches to trial design. In the traditional method of pre-specifying a fixed design and sample size, situations may arise when many participants may be exposed unnecessarily to toxic doses that are not efficacious. Adaptive designs that can address these limitations gained interest when noted in the 2004 Critical Path document issued by the FDA. The flexibility of the data-driven approach of adaptive trial designs allows for modifications of clinical trials based on the results of interim analyses. Despite differences among designs, there remain common factors that can enhance the efficiency of drug development to identify optimal dose groups through modification of the design based on interim results without detracting from the validity of the findings. A draft *Guidance for Industry* on adaptive trial designs is currently being prepared by the FDA. A draft "*Guidance for Industry* Non-Inferiority Clinical Trials" is available now on the FDA website at http://www.fda.gov/downloads/Drugs/GuidanceComplidanceRegulatoryInformation/Guidances/UCM202140.pdf

Safety evaluation

The therapeutic use of any drug entails risk. A safe drug product is one with a reasonable safety profile balanced with the expected benefit given the available alternatives. The primary goal of the review of the safety data is to identify major and common side effects (i.e., ADEs) to be weighed in risk-benefit assessments.

There are four main components to the safety evaluation in the target population. First and foremost, the FDA is especially interested in identifying "serious" events following drug use that may limit use of the new drug or require risk management procedures. Identification and characterization of serious drug experiences based on the evidence then ensues. A serious adverse event is one that results in: death, a life-threatening state, inpatient hospitalization, disability/incapacity, congenital anomaly/birth defect, or other important medical events. Other types of serious events include drug overdose, drug abuse, drug withdrawal, and failure of expected pharmacological action. In weighing the available body of evidence, the drug is deemed safe if the drug's potential for serious side effects (such as death or physical disability) is offset by the possibility of therapeutic benefit. Second, the reviewer estimates the frequency and severity of common adverse events. It is necessary to assess the adequacy of the safety data (including sufficient information) at the pertinent doses. In the confirmatory clinical trials, safety assessments such as vital signs, weight, laboratory measures, rating scales, electrocardiograms, and monitoring for reported and observed ADEs must be collected at baseline and appropriate follow-up times to identify the information for labeling needed to minimize or manage risks if necessary. Applicants are required also to provide safety updates to the FDA while the NDA is under review. Finally, unresolved safety concerns are identified in the review, including the amount of long-term data or insufficient data in specific populations such as children and adolescents.

Once serious ADEs are identified and characterized, in some cases the applicant may be required for approval to further evaluate and address serious risks in the post-marketing period. Additional studies of post-marketing safety may be proposed by the applicant in the NDA submission. If it is deemed to be necessary for approval to ensure that the benefits of a drug outweigh the risks beyond the information in labeling, the FDA may require that the applicant submit a Risk Evaluation and Mitigation Strategy (REMS) as part of the NDA. The REMS is a type of required risk management plan. The FDA may require the REMS to include one or more of the following elements that could affect a patient's decision to use or continue to use the drug product to help avoid serious adverse events:

- Medication Guide, which is a paper handout or pamphlet required to be distributed to patients with certain medications by the pharmacist;
- Patient Package Insert, which also provides drug safety labeling information;
- Communication plan, which may consist of letters or dissemination of information to healthcare practitioners to encourage implementation of clinical components or certain safety protocols; or
- Elements to assure safe use (ETASU), which usually serve in some way to restrict distribution of the drug.

Metrics are devised to assess the efficacy of the REMS in curbing the potential safety risk over time as well as delineation of a timetable for its assessment that is tailored to the drug's safety profile. The timetable for assessments must at minimum include assessments submitted to the FDA by 18 month, 3 year, and 7 year milestones after the REMS is initially approved to ensure that the potential benefits of the drug continue to outweigh the risks. For a list of approved REMS, visit http://www.fda.gov/Drugs/DrugSafety/PostmarketDrug-SafetyInformationforPatientsandProviders/ucm111350.htm

For Medication Guides, visit http://www.fda.gov/Drugs/DrugSafety/ucm085729.htm

Labeling

As the NDA review draws near completion, the labeling "negotiation process" comes to the forefront to reach agreement between the FDA and the applicant on final language. The interpretation of the data influencing regulatory decisions is affected by the uncertainty inherent in clinical research and different views on approaches to influencing clinical practice. Ultimately, the length of the negotiation process is determined in large part by the agency comments and the willingness of the applicant to reach agreement. In certain cases, the applicant will submit several iterations of labeling revisions before there is concurrence on labeling with the FDA. Agreement on final labeling language is required for approval.

Labeling provides the information on benefits and risk that is the basis for clinical decision-making. Labeling language is crafted to leave room for clinical judgment coupled with the patient's personal preferences. Each statement proposed by the applicant in drug labeling on key aspects such as patient population, drug in a class, dose, and timing must be supported by adequate data in the NDA. To protect patient safety, the evidentiary standard to incorporate safety data into labeling is lower than the threshold required for including efficacy claims. Arriving at the appropriate language in labeling is becoming more challenging in the wake of advancing science and technologies such as decisions arising about the incorporation of pharmacogenomics data. Consequently, past precedents do not necessarily predict future regulatory decision-making.

The Physician's Labeling Rule (PLR) issued in January 2006 has made labeling more user friendly and accessible to enhance safe and effective use of the drug product. The PLR labeling has three components: Highlights, Contents, and Full Prescribing Information. The Highlights of Prescribing Information section is the labeling tool that summarizes concisely up front the most important information for the prescribing healthcare provider. The contents depicted below are an index for the sections of the Full Prescribing Information.

Boxed Warning

1. Indications & Usage
2. Dosage & Administration
3. Dosage Forms & Strengths
4. Contraindications
5. Warnings & Precautions
6. Adverse Reactions
7. Drug Interactions
8. Use in Specific Populations
9. Drug Abuse & Dependence
10. Overdosage
11. Description
12. Clinical Pharmacology
13. Nonclinical Toxicology
14. Clinical Studies
15. References
16. How Supplied/Storage & Handling
17. Patient Counseling Information

The CONTRAINDICATIONS section of labeling comprises those rare scenarios in which the risk outweighs possible benefits of the drug and a causal link with the serious outcome has been established by exposure closely followed by the adverse drug reaction. Adverse drug experiences noted in the WARNINGS/PRECAUTIONS sections of labeling encompass safety issues observed with reasonable certainty of causality. Boxed WARNINGS are employed when adverse drug reactions are so serious that they must be highlighted in order to heighten awareness in the effort to reduce the risk of the adverse drug reaction. In the

ADVERSE REACTIONS section of labeling, events are included that are found in greater than or equal to 10% of the study drug group and twice the percentage in the placebo group. The PLR guidance suggests that only ADEs reasonably linked to the drug be included. Moreover, with the intent to prevent medication errors, product labels are reviewed by the FDA to identify and resolve issues of confused or mistaken identity that may arise in drug labeling.

New drug product labeling is catalogued now in an interagency clearinghouse for health information that provides the most current drug product information to patients and healthcare providers. Labeling can be accessed on this site through the National Library of Medicine at: http://dailymed.nlm.nih.gov.

The FDA's decision regarding approval is its ultimate risk-management action. If the NDA is deemed to meet the regulatory standards, the approval letter will be issued. If the FDA determines that it will not approve an application, a "complete response" letter will be issued. Complete response letters describe specific deficiencies for the applicant to address in a re-submission. Major reasons why an approval letter is not issued include inadequate data supporting safety and/or efficacy of the drug; evidence demonstrating the drug to be unsafe; or that manufacturing methods and controls do not suffice to preserve the identity, strength, quality, and purity of the drug product. The FDA provides the applicant with an opportunity for an end-of-review conference to discuss issues raised in the complete response letter. A new review cycle for the NDA starts on re-submission of an application addressing all deficiencies enumerated in the complete response letter.

The generic drug approval process

As a brand-name drug product nears patent expiration, generic drug manufacturers may file an application for approval to market a generic version of the drug. A generic drug product is comparable to the first approved drug that had been developed and manufactured by the pioneer pharmaceutical firm (also known as the reference listed drug [RLD] product) in terms of dosage form, strength, route of administration, quality performance characteristics, and intended use. The RLDs are identified in the FDA's list of Approved Drug Products with Therapeutic Equivalence Evaluations. ANDAs are submitted for approval to CDER's Office of Generic Drugs. In certain cases, suitability petitions are requests submitted to the FDA to permit filing of an ANDA for a drug that differs from the RLD product. If relevant, the applicant must have an approved suitability petition in order to file an ANDA with the proposed differences from the RLD.

Not surprisingly, the generic drug approval process is less intensive than the new drug process. There is no requirement for full reports on safety and effectiveness in ANDAs, as the safety and efficacy had already been demonstrated in the innovator's NDA for the approved drug product. The FDA requires, however, that the applicant establish that the generic copy works as well as the innovator drug through bioequivalence testing. Information in the bioequivalence review may include comparative dissolution testing for drugs with an established correlation between in vitro and in vivo effects and in vivo bioequivalence testing comparing the rate and extent of absorption of the generic to the reference drug product. The applicant provides data to ensure that the generic drug will be manufactured in a controlled, consistent manner. The manufacturing processes, material specifications and controls stability, sterilization procedures, and validation are reviewed to confirm that the drug will perform in an acceptable manner. Labeling for generic drug products is identical to the RLD labeling other than those differences attributed to change in drug manufacturer, patent or exclusivity information, or approval based on a suitability petition in which differences do not need additional evidence on safety or efficacy.

Once the ANDA is approved, the applicant manufactures and markets the generic version of the drug product. Approval of the first generic drug is rewarded by blocking approval of competitive ANDAs by other sponsors for 180 days of generics exclusivity. Were the ANDA to be approved prior to the expiration of patents or exclusivities attributed to the RLD, a tentative approval letter would be issued. Tentative approval does not allow the applicant to market the generic drug. The letter details the terms of the tentative approval of the generic drug product until the patent or exclusivity has expired.

Once a drug is approved, the primary responsibility for monitoring safety is that of healthcare providers and patients who make risk-benefit decisions tailored to each individual's profile. Together they are expected to use labeling information wisely to minimize risks while optimizing benefit.

Post-marketing drug regulation
Post-marketing surveillance

To monitor the safety of marketed drugs, the FDA maintains a complex system of post-marketing surveillance and risk-assessment systems to investigate the occurrence of serious and unexpected ADEs. The regulatory definition of "unexpected" is that ADEs are not listed in current labeling. The holder of the NDA must continue collection of safety data and review all ADE information obtained or otherwise received from any source. This surveillance system is important because large pre-marketing clinical trials cannot uncover every rare adverse event that may be observed once the drug is in wide use. This ongoing evaluation of drug safety over the lifecycle depends on recognition of adverse events and mandatory reporting by drug companies. This surveillance is complemented by the voluntary efforts of individuals to provide information on the occurrence and description of ADEs. Based on the ongoing evaluation of safety data, the FDA continues recommending ways to manage risk appropriately making use of a variety of systems and tools. Moreover, the FDA has a medical products reporting system called "MedWatch" to promote voluntary reporting of SAEs, medication errors, and drug product problems by patients and healthcare professionals: http://www.fda.gov/Safety/MedWatch/HowToReport/default.htm

The FDA's Adverse Event Reporting System (AERS) is an important drug safety tool. This computerized system combines and stores the reports of the voluntarily reported adverse drug events and medication errors from MedWatch as well as the required reports from manufacturers. These reports may form the basis of "signals" for potentially serious but unrecognized or uncharacterized ADEs and medication errors. The reports in AERS are evaluated by clinical safety reviewers in CDER to monitor and detect drug safety signals. The FDA conducts regular, bi-weekly screenings of AERS and posts a quarterly report on the FDA website. When a safety signal is identified, further testing is undertaken to characterize the association between drug use and the subsequent adverse event. The hypothetical association may be evaluated using various epidemiological and analytic databases, studies, and other resources when appropriate. When new safety information that appears clinically important emerges, the FDA may take regulatory actions with the goal of improving product safety.

The FDA is especially interested in keeping healthcare professionals informed about new and emerging safety concerns. The agency may issue a communication to the public describing the safety concern in the interest of informing physicians, other healthcare providers, and patients. In these communications, the FDA usually shares information on the safety issue, in addition to factors to consider when making treatment decisions, and other clinical information that patients need to know in order to safely use the drug. The FDA's information sharing is mainly accomplished through MedWatch Safety Alerts: http://www.fda.gov/Safety/MedWatch/SafetyInformation/default.htm and other FDA safety web postings. New safety information, such as potential new safety risks, is posted on the FDA website in a quarterly report.

The Food and Drug Administration Amendments Act (FDAAA)

FDAAA gives new authorities to the FDA to require manufacturers to conduct necessary post-approval studies and clinical trials to assess known safety risks related to use of the drug product, to evaluate signals of serious risk related to use of the drug, or to identify an unexpected serious risk when the available data indicate such potential. There are numerous types of post-marketing requirements (PMRs) including, though not limited to, clinical studies, safety studies in animals, in vitro laboratory safety studies, pharmacokinetics studies, or drug interaction evaluations. A clinical PMR could be a deferred pediatric study, a condition of accelerated approval, or a safety study or trial that a sponsor is required to conduct after approval. The condition that a PMR will be undertaken to explore a potential safety signal is sometimes necessary for approval. A PMR can also be imposed post-approval. In contrast, a post-marketing commitment (PMC) is a study to be conducted that the applicant agrees in writing to conduct following approval. The PMC, though, is not required by law. The FDA monitors the progress of PMRs and PMCs to ensure timely completion.

The FDA developed a website also with post-marketing drug safety information for patients and providers to improve transparency, which is available at http://www.fda.gov/Drugs/DrugSafety/PostmarketDrugSafetyInformationforPatientsandProviders/default.htm. The FDA is required to post information from each summary analysis of ADEs received for newly approved drugs. These summary reports are prepared after a drug has been approved for 18 months or after 10 000 individuals have used the drug, whichever is later. The summary report must include the identification of any new risks not previously identified, potential new risks, or known risks reported in unusually high numbers. FDAAA mandates that the FDA conduct regular, bi-weekly screening of the Adverse Event Reporting System and post a quarterly report on the system website. The FDA now posts on the internet a quarterly report of new safety information or potential signals of serious risk identified from AERS. The presence of a drug on this list does not mean that the FDA has concluded that the drug has the listed risk. It conveys that the FDA has identified a potential safety issue to explore.

The FDA established the Drug Safety Oversight Board in 2005, which is composed of members of government from FDA and other agencies under Health and Human Services. The Board's primary objectives are to offer independent oversight and advice to CDER leadership on the management of important drug safety issues and the flow of emerging safety information to healthcare professionals and patients. An important drug safety issue for the Board is one that would alter the balance of benefit to risk in such a way as to affect decisions about prescribing or taking the drug.

A number of noteworthy scientific and regulatory advances that influence drug development are emerging. The Sentinel System is the FDA's national electronic surveillance system being developed and implemented in stages as the science and technology evolve. As currently envisioned, the FDA would utilize active surveillance methodologies to monitor post-marketing medical product safety. The system is a distributed model in which all personally identifiable information remains in its local environment, protected by existing firewalls and managed by those most familiar with the data. The FDA targets safety questions regarding drug products with associated ADEs to develop for submission to data holders, including academic centers, healthcare systems, and medical insurance companies. Participating data holders evaluate the adverse events associated with the target drugs in their databases and only provide summaries of the results. The Sentinel Initiative is expected to complement available methods for safety signal identification in several ways to:

- improve capability to identify and evaluate safety issues in near real time;
- expand capacity for evaluating safety issues;
- improve access to longer-term data;
- improve access to defined populations (e.g., the elderly, patients with diabetes);
- improve identification of increased risk of common adverse events (e.g., myocardial infarction, fracture) that healthcare practitioners may not suspect are related to medical products.

The "Safe Use" initiative is the term coined by the FDA describing the long-term effort to expand the Agency's mission to ensure that medicines are used safely and as indicated throughout the drug's lifecycle. This initiative is accomplished by working in partnership with other components of the healthcare system.

Recent developments in the pharmacogenomics arena are promising. A guidance titled "Pharmacogenomic Data Submissions" (2005) signaled the FDA's willingness to review submitted exploratory pharmacogenomic data not otherwise required for regulatory decision-making classified as "voluntary genomic data submissions". One basic area being explored actively is the need to develop consensus standards for exchanging and presenting genomic drug development data.

Summary

The reader should appreciate now that the FDA's regulatory process strives to maintain a challenging balance intended to foster innovation in drug development while attempting to manage or even minimize safety risks. The foremost pillar of the new drug approval process is adequate and well-controlled clinical trial testing of safety and efficacy in the population for the intended use. A dynamic confluence of scientific, medical, technological, and policy factors interact with a growing framework of laws that shape the process of drug development and regulation. Labeling has been given considerable emphasis because it is the chief vehicle that the FDA and the manufacturer use to communicate risk and benefit to the public for optimal use of drugs.

Suggested reading

Hamburg, M. A. and Sharfstein, J. M. (2009). The FDA as a Public Health Agency. *New Engl J Med*, 360 (24), 2493–5.

Piantadosi, S. (1997). *Clinical Trials: A Methodologic Perspective*. New York: John Wiley & Sons.

Woodcock, J. (2009). A difficult balance – pain management, drug safety, and the FDA. *New Engl J Med*, 361 (22), 2105–7.

FDA Website

Supporting information:

http://www.fda.gov/cder/regulatory

The U.S. Food and Drug Administration (2004). Innovation/Stagnation, Challenge and Opportunity on the Critical Path to New Medical Products. March 2004.

Draft Guidance for Industry: Format and Content of Proposed Risk Evaluation and Mitigation Strategies (REMS). REMS Assessments and Proposed REMS Modifications.

General Accounting Office report, FDA Drug Approval: Review Time Has Decreased in Recent Years, http://www.fda.gov/AboutFDA/ReportsManualsForms/Reports/UserFeeReports/PerformanceReports/PDUFA/ucm117257.htm

The views are those of the author and not necessarily those of the Food and Drug Administration.

Essential CNS drug development – pre-clinical development

Alan J. Cross and Frank D. Yocca

Introduction

Neuropsychiatric disorders generally involve a complex interaction of genetic and environmental factors, leading to heterogeneity in terms of symptom presentation and treatment responsiveness. In addition many disorders follow a chronic path of relapse and remission which is also highly variable, unpredictable, and poorly understood. In most cases our knowledge of pathophysiology is limited and most therapeutic approaches focus on treating symptoms rather than underlying mechanisms of illness. Given the chronic recurrent nature of many neuropsychiatric disorders, symptomatic treatments often involve prolonged drug administration and a requirement for stringent demands in terms of long-term safety and tolerability. All of these factors contribute to the enormous challenge of discovering and developing novel drug candidates for neuropsychiatric illness (see Panagalos *et al.*, 2007, for discussion). Despite this complexity, new treatments for neuropsychiatric disorders continue to bring benefit to patients and novel approaches continue to emerge; however, progress has been slow and considerable patient need remains. Indeed, few neuropsychiatric disorders can be considered to have anything close to satisfactory treatment.

Serendipity is often acknowledged as playing a major role in CNS drug discovery. Whether it is really serendipity or rather astute clinical observation remains a matter of debate. It is, however, clear that historically the majority of successful truly novel approaches have relied heavily on the ability of physicians to detect therapeutic effects rather than on a mechanism-based rational approach to drug discovery. The tremendous advances in understanding disease biology following recent investments into basic and clinical neuroscience (the decade of the brain) will hopefully provide the foundation for discovering and developing new therapies for CNS disorders based on such a rational approach to drug discovery.

The drug discovery process

The drug discovery process is often depicted as a linear progression from identification of a drug target through to development of the drug candidate (Figure 1). We can define the drug target as the molecular site of action of the drug, and we can consider a drug target fully validated when clinical efficacy has been demonstrated by several agents active at the target in pivotal efficacy studies. Whilst this process provides a useful framework for

Essential CNS Drug Development, ed. A. Kalali, Sheldon Preskorn, J. Kwentus, and Stephen M. Stahl. Published by Cambridge University Press. © Cambridge University Press 2012.

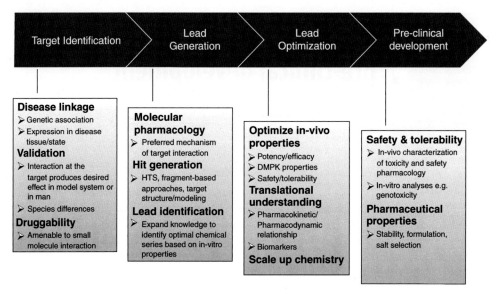

Figure 1. Drug discovery process.

organizing the complex multidisciplinary activities involved in drug discovery, many programs will deviate from a simple linear process and there are indeed many successful drugs which have been developed without following this simple model.

The process can be divided into four phases; each phase consists of many interrelated activities, the key components of which are outlined in the boxes in Figure 1. The process is depicted as starting with identification of the appropriate molecular target; once the target is clearly defined the next step is to identify lead compounds (lead generation) with the appropriate properties to support a medicinal chemistry (lead optimization) effort. Once the properties have been optimized, drug candidates are characterized during the pre-clinical development phase with respect to their safety, tolerability, and efficacy.

The number and diversity of targets currently exploited in the major neuropsychiatric disorders are extremely limited, and only a few new targets have found utility in recent years. It has been estimated that the total number of clinically validated drug targets is between 200 and 300, and of these, CNS drugs exploit fewer than 20 (Imming *et al.*, 2006; Overington *et al.*, 2006). Indeed as mentioned previously, the major classes of CNS drugs exploit a limited number of monoamine transporters, GPCRs, enzymes, and ion channels. There is thus a very high premium placed on the identification and validation of new drug targets in the treatment of neuropsychiatric disorders. Underlying this, many novel approaches have been taken to clinical testing without generating compelling efficacy or demonstrating advantage over currently available treatments. There has thus been a shift in focus in both industry and academia away from target identification towards the translation and validation of novel targets for the treatment of neuropsychiatric disorders. Whilst there is a renewed focus on "picking the right target" it should be kept in mind that many compounds fail in development for reasons other than lack of efficacy. Generating candidates with good safety and tolerability combined with the need to gain access to the central nervous system puts an additional premium on the so-called "druggability" of molecules. The diversity of chemical structures and approaches employed to overcome these barriers has increased dramatically and is now complemented with the emerging promise of biopharmaceuticals.

The technological advances in molecular neuropharmacology and structural biology and the potential of large molecule therapeutics increase the number of potential drug targets and the ways in which these targets can be addressed to design novel therapeutic agents for CNS disorders. It is hoped that when combined with a rational approach to target identification based on the understanding of pathophysiological mechanisms, we will witness a new generation of CNS therapeutics bringing real benefit to patients.

Identifying CNS drug targets
Reverse pharmacology and multi-target agents

Given that most novel treatments are based on serendipitous clinical observation, it is not surprising that most targets for neuropsychiatric drugs have been derived through pharmacological understanding of the mechanism of action of known agents. As these treatments are primarily symptomatic, it follows that the targets for these drugs are all involved in neuronal signaling and neurotransmitter mechanisms. A historically successful approach has been to identify the mechanism of action of known therapeutic agents and modify the pharmacology to produce better-tolerated agents. This approach, sometimes called reverse pharmacology, has been the mainstay of drug discovery in psychiatry, although it is debatable how much additional benefit can be extracted from the currently available targets. More recently it has been proposed that defined combinations of pharmacological activity (multi-target therapeutics) may offer additional advantages (Zimmerman et al., 2007). Within the realm of monoamine reuptake inhibitors as antidepressants, the initial reverse pharmacology approach drove towards increasingly selective inhibitors of serotonin transporters (SSRIs). As more SSRIs became available, the need to produce additional benefit focused drug discovery efforts on the development of dual serotonin-noradrenaline reuptake inhibitors (SNRIs) or even triple reuptake inhibitors including dopamine reuptake inhibition. Given the structural similarities between the different monoamine reuptake transporters, and also between their natural substrates, it is perhaps not surprising that drug candidates can be identified with differential activity at these targets. Although it has been possible to identify compounds with broader multi-target pharmacology, it is not clear whether this can be achieved in a rational predictive manner or whether we are still relying on serendipity. If the desired multi-target pharmacologies are associated with structurally distinct target binding sites (pharmacophores), for example at both a GPCR and a transporter, the rational design of such agents becomes increasingly unpredictable (see Paolini et al., 2006, for discussion).

The example in Figure 2 depicts the development of dopamine D2 receptor antagonists derived from the initial clinical finding of the antipsychotic efficacy of the phenothiazine chlorpromazine. Although phenothiazines have a broad activity at many monoamine receptors, clinical and pre-clinical pharmacological studies suggested that dopamine D2 antagonist activity was the only prerequisite for antipsychotic activity. This hypothesis was supported by the subsequent development of selective D2 antagonists such as the substituted benzamides, which retained antipsychotic activity. The development of antipsychotic drugs based

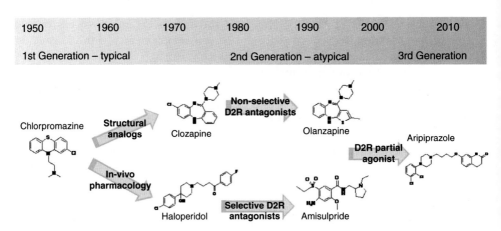

Figure 2. Reverse pharmacology – the mainstay of target discovery in CNS disorders.

on this principle has been extended by building in additional pharmacological activities (a multi-target approach) or by generating partial agonists (exemplified by aripiprazole) to improve the tolerability and efficacy profile.

The target class approach

A further extension of this approach has been to search for novel structurally related targets within a particular target family or class, for example G-protein-coupled receptors (see Heilker *et al.*, 2009, for discussion). GPCRs form one of the most abundant target classes in the human genome and are an important target class for CNS active drugs. The target family approach began by exploiting functionally related targets, for example the family of serotonin receptors, but then expanded to include all members of a particular target family. Complementing this approach is the concept that certain target classes are more favorable (i.e. druggable) than others in terms of our ability to identify drug-like molecules which interact with the target. Whilst an array of target classes have found utility in the broad realm of drug discovery, the range of targets currently available in CNS disorders is limited and GPCRs remain the predominant target family.

As depicted in Figure 3, the majority of CNS drugs modulate neurotransmitter systems involved in synaptic transmission. Important CNS drugs target many components of this process, but the most commonly exploited targets are cell-surface proteins such as GPCRs, sodium-dependent monoamine transporters, and ligand-gated ion channels.

The target class approach has generated a large number of potential targets; however, as discussed earlier, success is dependent on our ability to select and validate the correct target. This has proven particularly difficult with so-called orphan GPCRs; whilst many of these have been successfully de-orphanized, few have been functionally validated and led to the discovery of good drug candidates.

An interesting example of this approach is MCH-1 receptor for melanocyte concentrating hormone (MCH). MCH is a neuropeptide initially identified in frogs and subsequently in rodents in the hypothalamic pituitary system. MCH regulates feeding behavior and has more recently been shown to modulate "mood" and reward in animals. The identity of the MCH receptor was unknown until it was found to be an orphan GPCR

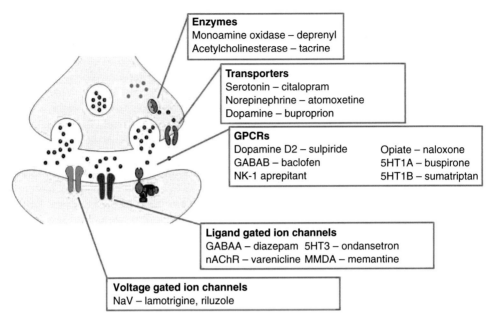

Figure 3. The major target classes exploited by current CNS drugs.

known as SLC-1 or GPR24. The identification of SLC-1 as the MCH-1 receptor followed two related approaches, both starting with the expression of SLC-1 in recombinant systems.

- SLC-1 was expressed in cell lines to generate a functional assay, and tissue extracts were added to these cells to induce a biological response. The active component of these tissue extracts was isolated and characterized as MCH.
- The second approach involved using a collection of pharmacologically active substances to activate the recombinant receptor. Of those compounds found to be effective only MCH was a naturally occurring ligand.

The identification of the MCH-1 receptor opened the way for drug discovery efforts focused initially on the central control of food intake. The role of MCH in food intake was known; knowledge of the receptor and the central sites of action of MCH in this context were established. It was later found that the receptor was present in areas involved not only in feeding but also in neuronal circuits involved in reward/anhedonia. The discovery of the receptor and identification of the natural ligand supported the development of high-throughput screening assays and the generation of drug-like CNS active MCH-1 antagonists. Interestingly these antagonists are active in models of food intake and are also active in animal models of anxiolytic and antidepressant-like activity. Currently several MCH antagonists are in clinical development for the treatment of obesity and depression.

This type of approach has extended beyond GPCRs to encompass most of the major target classes. Novel members of many target classes have been identified; for example, within the transporters, novel family members identified from genomics include transporters for neurotransmitter amino acids and biogenic amines (Krishnamurthy *et al.*, 2009).

To date none of these have been clinically validated; however, novel drugs acting at previously unidentified amino acid and biogenic amine targets are in clinical development. More success has been found within the ligand-gated ion channel family, either through the identification of specific receptor subtypes or through novel members of a particular family; again novel drugs are in development for several of these targets. Voltage-gated ion channels are a large superfamily with many subfamilies of potential targets. Voltage-gated ion channels are the targets of many anticonvulsants and analgesic drugs; however, a lack of good pharmacological tools with reasonable selectivity has hindered the validation of selected ion channels in relation to specific disorders. Genetic studies have implicated a range of potassium and sodium channels in inherited forms of epilepsy and sensory disorders. Combined with phenotypic studies of knockout mice, it is likely that voltage-gated ion channels, and in particular potassium channels (Wulff et al., 2009), will have great potential as targets for the treatment of CNS disorders. On the other hand, several features limit the feasibility of identifying selective drug-like molecules acting at these targets. In general voltage-gated ion channels are complex multimeric proteins which are difficult to express and assess functionally in screening assays and it has proven difficult to generate compounds with the required selectivity.

It is clear that a thematic approach based on established target families can provide a source of novel targets with potential utility. Although these are from so-called druggable families the success of finding good drug-like molecules acting at these targets has not been uniformly high, and many interesting targets have resisted pharmacological exploitation. For example the GABA$_B$ receptor, a member of the family III GPCRs, has been considered a highly attractive CNS target which has so far resisted many attempts to identify drug-like antagonists.

It is worth noting that several target classes which have been widely exploited outside CNS indication have proven problematic in terms of drug discovery in CNS disorders. It is noteworthy that kinases (one of the largest target families) are currently devoid of CNS active drugs; similarly nuclear hormone receptors have been difficult to exploit. Whilst these are clearly druggable in a generic sense, several factors which are important in the CNS context limit feasibility, in particular the ability to access intracellular targets whilst maintaining good CNS exposure.

Mechanism-based approaches

Considerable progress has been made in exploiting an understanding of disease pathophysiology to identify novel targets for the treatment of neurodegenerative disorders. Identifying the selective vulnerability of dopamine neurons in Parkinson's disease led to the development of l-dopa as a replacement therapy; similarly acetylcholinesterase inhibitors were introduced to the treatment of Alzheimer's disease based on a selective loss of cholinergic neurons.

Alzheimer's disease also represents a useful example of a mechanism-based approach to potentially disease-modifying treatments within CNS disorders. The combination of genetics and molecular pathology has contributed to an understanding of the role of amyloid production in the pathogenesis of Alzheimer's disease and several drug targets have been identified in this pathway.

The amyloid hypothesis is based on the critical involvement of β-amyloid in AD pathogenesis (Figure 4). Amyloid Aβ peptides are the main components of amyloid plaques

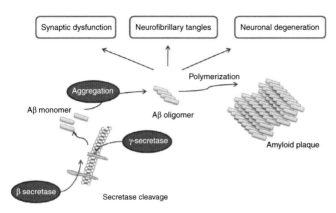

Figure 4. The amyloid hypothesis of Alzheimer's disease as a basis for target identification. The initial finding that the pathological hallmark of Alzheimer's disease, amyloid plaques, are formed from a self-aggregating Aβ peptide, which is in turn a product of cleavage of the amyloid precursor protein APP, forms a cornerstone of the amyloid hypothesis. In addition, mutations altering the enzymic activity of a proteolytic enzyme complex (γ-secretase) involved in cleavage of the APP or polymorphisms in the APP gene itself have been found to be responsible for some forms of familial Alzheimer's disease. This forms another foundation for the hypothesis, and highlights γ-secretase as a potential drug target in this process. β-Secretase, the other enzyme identified in Aβ peptide synthesis, is another potential target of intense interest. Other points of intervention in the process include amyloid aggregation inhibitors, which bind to Aβ peptides to prevent oligomerization, or Aβ peptide removal primarily by sequestration by means of active or passive immunization. The hypothesis is of particular interest in CNS drug discovery as it is one of the first pathophysiological mechanisms to be deciphered at the molecular level; however, a critical test of the hypothesis in the clinic has yet to be completed.

and are derived from a larger amyloid precursor protein by proteolytic cleavage. Amyloid Aβ peptides, in particular Aβ 1–42, are hypothesized to be responsible for the neuronal and synaptic toxicity characteristic of AD. Several lines of evidence support this hypothesis. Genetic studies have shown that mutations in APP or presenilin are associated with familial AD. Presenilin has been shown to be a catalytic subunit of γ-secretase, one of the enzymes involved in APP cleavage to yield Aβ peptides. Disease-associated mutations in either APP or presenilin result in over-production of amyloidogenic Aβ peptides. Transgenic mice over-expressing these mutations produce plaques reminiscent of AD plaques, and synaptic dysfunction. Based on this hypothesis, several targets in the amyloid Aβ pathway have been identified, most notably γ-secretase and β-secretase, the proteolytic enzymes involved in the production of Aβ peptides.

A further approach to disease modification in AD is based on the observation in transgenic mice that passive or active immunization to Aβ peptides results in a reduction of plaque load, and recent preliminary clinical studies suggest this may also occur in AD patients. These approaches are not without risk; in particular, γ-secretase cleaves a multitude of substrates involved in normal cellular functioning. In addition, immunization approaches have been associated with the risk of cerebral hemorrhage although some evidence suggests that passive immunization with monoclonal antibodies to defined Aβ epitopes may avoid this risk. Despite these concerns, several of these approaches are currently in pivotal efficacy studies and are expected to readout in the near future, providing the first data on the validity of the amyloid hypothesis (Citron, 2010).

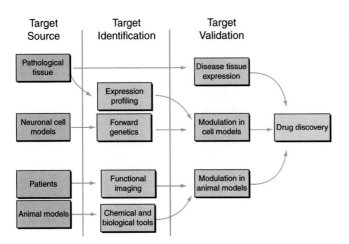

Figure 5. Target identification and validation in CNS disorders.

Much has been made of the lack of success in applying molecular pharmacology, genomics, and genetics to the discovery of new targets for drug treatment in psychiatry (see Agid *et al.*, 2007, for discussion). One reason for the lack of success has been a lack of mechanistic understanding of disease biology to provide a framework for target validation. The advances in neuroimaging, functional morphology, and genetics of the last 5–10 years have begun to generate new understanding of disease mechanisms in terms of aberrant neuronal circuitry in relation to certain symptoms. Moreover, as our understanding of these mechanisms grows, so the development of more relevant disease models can advance. Within this context, mechanisms can be seen as relating to function and dysfunction in neural circuits underlying behaviors and traits common to neuropsychiatric disorders (Spedding *et al.*, 2005), rather than the biochemical pathology often associated with neurodegenerative disorders.

A rational approach to target identification (shown in Figure 5) can be based either on molecular pathology (as in the previous example of Alzheimer's disease) or on a systems-based mechanistic approach (as in the example of schizophrenia; Figure 6). Precise knowledge of molecular pathology allows the use of cellular models and molecular tools to validate concepts. With a systems-based approach, more reliance is placed on animal models and the use of pharmacological tools to provide initial validation (based on Lindsay, 2003).

Target validation in pre-clinical CNS drug discovery

Target validation involves two components: demonstrating a connection or involvement of a target with a disease process, and demonstrating that drug interaction with the target or modulation of the target modifies the disease process (Knowles and Gromo, 2003). During the drug discovery process, target validation can be performed initially using in vitro or in vivo models but ultimately relies on demonstrating a clinical effect in patients.

Confidence in validation during the discovery process is critically dependent on the validity of the cellular or animal models available. Some aspects of neurodegenerative

Schizophrenia

- Schematic of Glutamate Hypothesis

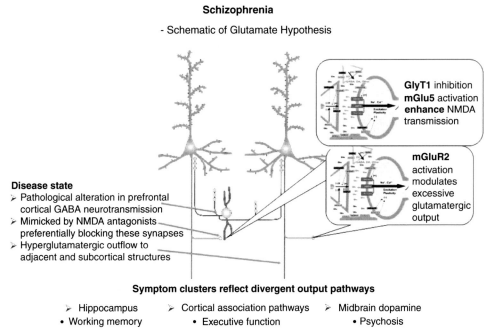

GlyT1 inhibition
mGlu5 activation
enhance NMDA
transmission

mGluR2
activation
modulates
excessive
glutamatergic
output

Disease state
➢ Pathological alteration in prefrontal
   cortical GABA neurotransmission
➢ Mimicked by NMDA antagonists
   preferentially blocking these synapses
➢ Hyperglutamatergic outflow to
   adjacent and subcortical structures

Symptom clusters reflect divergent output pathways

| ➢ Hippocampus | ➢ Cortical association pathways | ➢ Midbrain dopamine |
| • Working memory | • Executive function | • Psychosis |

Figure 6. Systems-based approach to drug discovery in psychiatry. See plate section for color version.

disorders such as Alzheimer's disease and Parkinson's disease can be modeled in in vitro systems based on the molecular pathology of these disorders. These systems are attractive in that they enable some degree of confidence in the target to be obtained early in the discovery process. In addition, tool compounds and biological reagents which may not be useful for in vivo use can be used with in vitro systems. In Alzheimer's disease, over-production of Aβ can be modeled in a variety of recombinant and native cells. Such systems have been used extensively to demonstrate the effectiveness of secretase inhibitors for preventing the production of amyloidogenic peptides. It is generally assumed that tests based on intact native neurons are preferable to recombinant systems; however, the availability of such systems is extremely limited particularly with respect to human cells. Although the use of inducible pluripotent stem cells carries considerable promise in this regard, much remains to be done to establish this approach.

Use of animal models in CNS drug discovery

Whilst in vitro approaches have been used extensively to identify and gain initial validation of targets, considerably more emphasis has been placed on the use of animal models. For most neuropsychiatric disorders it has proven extremely difficult to model disease-relevant pathophysiological and behavioral phenotypes in experimental animals. Given the dramatic differences in structure, functional morphology, and behavioral repertoire it is of course impossible to model the entire spectrum of neuropsychiatric illness in experimental animals. Despite this, animal models have provided critical information in terms of modeling aspects of disease and in modeling CNS drug action. In this regard it is important to consider the validity of animal models with regard to their purpose; for example, a model designed to mimic certain aspects of symptomatology may be quite different from a model designed to study the effects of therapeutic agents. Three main factors can be considered in terms of the validity of animal models, the relevance of which will depend upon the purpose of the model.

- Construct validity. This is generally defined as the accuracy with which the animal model reflects the disease process. Closely related to this is the concept of etiological validity, which relates to the similarity between the etiology of the disease and the conditions of the model. For example, using a genetic manipulation identical to a causative genetic change in human illness to produce an animal model would be of high construct validity. Conversely, modeling psychiatric illness, where pathophysiology is poorly understood, is considerably more problematic.

- Face validity. This can be defined as the similarity in the phenomenology of the model compared to the human disease. With regard to models based on neuropathological change, such as the degeneration of dopaminergic neurons in models of Parkinson's disease, the similarity of the degenerative process relative to the degeneration in Parkinson's disease would be a key factor. This becomes more complex in cases where certain aspects of behavior are being modeled. In most cases objective measures of behaviors are difficult to obtain, and even in cases where more objective measures can be made, the mechanisms underlying behavioral outcomes can be difficult to establish.

- Predictive validity. This is generally defined as the ability of a model to predict the human outcome, for example, whether the outcome of the drug effect in the animal models parallels the outcome in patients. In psychiatry many models exist that are designed to predict therapeutic effects of drugs, and whilst these may have some predictive value in terms of mechanism, they tend to have very low construct and face validity. Often these models are validated with drugs of known therapeutic benefit, and it is unclear whether this predictive capacity will translate to novel drug mechanisms.

In Alzheimer's disease, two approaches to animal modeling are of interest: disease modification (Philipson *et al.*, 2010) and cognition enhancement (Sarter, 2006). Transgenic mice expressing familial AD mutations have generated animal models reproducing several of the pathological features of AD. Transgenic mice expressing normal human APP do not produce amyloid deposits unless very high levels of expression are used. In contrast, mice expressing APP with disease-associated mutations produce amyloid deposits at lower expression levels. Mice expressing APP or PS mutations, often in combination, are some of the most frequently used transgenic models and display AD-like pathology, including Aβ deposition and cerebrovascular amyloid. At this stage it is clear that such models lack some of the key features of the disease. It has been difficult to describe a reliable behavioral phenotype which shows progressive deterioration in response to Aβ accumulation in these animals. Neuronal degeneration (certainly with the pattern associated with AD) has also not been shown, although synaptic dysfunction may be present. Thus testing of secretase inhibitors in these animals is limited to the use of Aβ peptide production (essentially a pharmacodynamic marker) and it is unknown by how much Aβ peptide levels need to be reduced, and for how long, to translate into meaningful clinical benefit in patients. The use of more sophisticated transgenic models may address some of these issues (see Philipson *et al.*, 2010, for discussion).

A second type of model focuses on the cognitive deficits of Alzheimer's disease. Based on the selective loss of cholinergic neurons in Alzheimer's disease, lesions of cholinergic neurons, pharmacological antagonists, or aged animals have been used to assess cognitive deficits. None of these replicate the pathological changes seen in AD and thus construct validity is restricted. These manipulations have been produced in a variety of species including nonhuman primates and to a varying extent replicate some of the cognitive deficits associated with Alzheimer's disease. The predictive validity of these models varies considerably and is mainly assessed by the generation of false positives, as the only validated approaches to cognition enhancement in Alzheimer's disease are cholinesterase inhibitors and NMDA antagonists.

In psychiatry, animal models have relied heavily on demonstrating behavioral effects of known therapeutic agents with little construct or face validity (Arguello and Gogos, 2006). More recently focus has shifted towards animal models of particular defined features or intermediate phenotypes of psychiatric illness including behavioral and functional imaging measures. Given the tremendous differences in structure and complexity of rodent brain compared to human brain, it is extremely difficult to model even defined components of complex human behavior in animals. However, progress has been made in modeling specific behavioral intermediate phenotypes in animals (Gould and Gottesman, 2006; Meyer-Lindenberg and Weinberger, 2006) and linking them to defined neuronal pathways and mechanisms. The predictive capacity of this approach, whilst intuitively attractive, has yet to be established in a clinical treatment setting.

Target validation tools

A variety of tools are available for pre-clinical target validation and have been successfully applied in CNS drug discovery. Traditionally, chemical or pharmacological tools have been used to probe target function. Whilst small molecule pharmacological tools have the advantage of ease of use in animal models, pharmacological selectivity and brain exposure are critical factors. For novel targets, generating good pharmacological tools can be a difficult and time-consuming process. In many cases such tools are not available before a considerable investment in medicinal chemistry has been made.

Increasingly, biological tools such as antibodies, interference RNA etc. have been used along with genetic manipulations to gain early target validation in the absence of good small molecule tools. Whilst this offers the advantage of higher throughput and specificity, delivery to the intact CNS remains a key issue, particularly if behavioral analysis is the endpoint in such validation experiments.

Generating lead compounds
The concept of druggability in CNS drug discovery

The probability of being able to interact with and modulate the target with a small molecule drug is often referred to as druggability (Cheng *et al.*, 2007; Schmidtke and Barril, 2010). Determining a target's druggability experimentally is costly and time-consuming and considerable effort has been put into predicting druggability in silico. As mentioned earlier, druggability can be estimated by classifying targets into gene

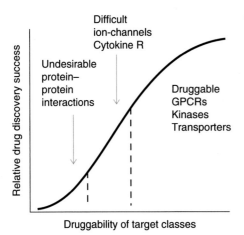

Figure 7. The concept of druggability. This was initially based on simple assumptions of particular target families being amenable to small molecule interactions. More recently, attempts have been made to generate empirical data based on low-affinity binding of molecular fragments, combined with sophisticated modeling algorithms to produce more predictive data. Whilst these concepts have been widely applied in a generic sense, specific application to CNS targets has been less extensively studied.

families which have previously been shown to be druggable. More recently, structural information on target binding sites and physicochemical properties have been used to create predictive algorithms (Figure 7).

The discovery and refinement of lead compounds is an extremely complex and time-consuming undertaking. Within the context of CNS drug discovery, this task is even more complicated due to the additional constraints required to ensure adequate exposure in the brain and by the requirements for safety and tolerability supporting prolonged treatment periods. An industrial-scale approach to the discovery of novel chemical starting points involves the use of high-throughput screening technologies combined with large collections (libraries) of diverse chemical compounds. Screening technologies have generally involved considerable miniaturization of assays using recombinant systems combined with robotics and micro-fluidics (Wu and Doberstein, 2006). These approaches have been successfully applied in many cases, and have been refined by supplementing compound libraries with information generated using in silico screens and informatics. Whilst these methods have been effective, it is now apparent that a more refined approach based on knowledge of the target structure, molecular pharmacology, and signaling mechanisms may be a more productive way to lead generation, particularly with regard to CNS targets (Babaoglu and Shiochet, 2006; Jorgensen, 2009).

Several examples of how this interaction between lead generation chemistry and molecular pharmacology are worth considering in the context of CNS drug discovery with different types of target and approach (see Heilker *et al.*, 2009, for discussion of techno-logical aspects).

In the example of β-secretase, high-throughput screening approaches failed to produce viable drug-like starting points to support a chemical synthesis program. Application of a fragment-based approach coupled with knowledge of the target structure and active site generated potent drug-like inhibitors with novel chemistry (Figure 8).

G-protein-coupled receptors

The GPCR superfamily contains more than 1200 members, broadly divided into three major classes which differ markedly in their structure, the nature of their natural ligands, and their signaling properties. The majority fall within family 1, and are receptors for neurotransmitter amines, peptides, and lipids. In general, the binding sites of the natural

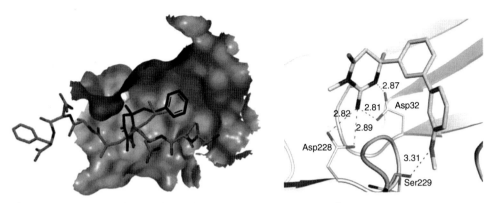

Figure 8. Fragment-based approaches to lead generation. See plate section for color version.

ligands are readily amenable to small molecule medicinal chemistry and have been extensively exploited as CNS drug targets.

Family 1 GPCRs are composed of a single domain of seven transmembrane α-helices which contain the ligand binding pocket. In the case of these receptors, the binding pocket is formed as a crevice between the transmembrane helices and has evolved to bind the small polar ligands which are the natural agonists. Given the similarity in the chemical properties of the endogenous ligands, it is not surprising that a high degree of overlap occurs between the different amine receptor pharmacophores. Thus identifying drug-like compounds with a high degree of selectivity for one particular amine receptor has proven extremely difficult; nevertheless highly selective compounds acting at the most promiscuous GPCRs have been described. Other members of the family 1 receptors include cannabinoid receptors in subfamily I, the tachykinin receptors in subfamily II, and the opioid receptors in subfamily IV.

The family 2 receptors contain a number of important CNS targets, including the CRF-1 receptor. Family 2 receptors contain a large N-terminal ecto-domain which plays an important role in agonist binding. Peptide agonists are thought to bind to the receptor in a two-step process. Binding occurs initially to the extracellular domain, which facilitates a binding to a second site in or close to the transmembrane domain. Binding to the transmembrane domain induces a confirmation or activation of the receptor, leading to G-protein complex recruitment and intracellular signal transduction. Whilst some peptide antagonists of binding to the extracellular domain have been described, most small molecule antagonists do not bind to this site, but bind to a distinct allosteric site within the transmembrane domain. Binding of small molecule allosteric antagonists within this site is thought to stabilize an inactive state of the receptor.

The family 3 GPCRs contain only about 25 members, including the metabotropic glutamate receptors and the GABA$_B$ receptors. These receptors contain a very large extracellular domain, which encompasses the agonist binding site. In general, family 3 receptors form dimers which are required for active receptor function. Agonist binding induces a large confirmation or change in the extracellular domain (often called a Venus fly trap mechanism) which is translated through changes in the transmembrane domain to G-protein activation. Given the nature of the endogenous ligands, the agonist binding site is not generally considered to be amenable to drugs with good CNS properties. However, as with family 2 receptors, allosteric sites have been identified in the transmembrane domain which bear similarity to the agonist binding site family 1 receptors.

Ion channels

Membrane-bound ion channels represent a ubiquitously expressed series of multimeric proteins, involved in the regulation of membrane potential, neuronal plasticity, and neurotransmitter release, which are well-precedented targets for CNS drugs. Voltage-gated ion channels are regulated by membrane potential and can be further characterized on the basis of ionic permeability and the kinetics of their channel properties. Ligand-gated ion channels are modulated by the binding of endogenous ligand to change the conductance properties or voltage dependence of the channel.

The fast inhibitory synaptic interactions of GABA are mediated by the $GABA_A$ receptor, the prototypic ligand-gated ion channel. The $GABA_A$ receptor belongs to a family of pentameric ion channels which includes nicotinic acetylcholine receptors and the ionotropic glutamate receptors. The $GABA_A$ receptor can comprise potentially 16 different subunits, five of which subunits are arranged around a central core forming the ion channel. Each subunit has a large N-terminal domain which extends into the extracellular space, and contributes to the agonist binding site. Although a plethora of possible combinations of subunits exist, in general $GABA_A$ receptors are composed of two alpha, two beta, and a gamma subunit (see Whiting, 2003, for review). Binding of GABA to the receptor modulates chloride flux through the ion channel, hyperpolarizing membrane potential and inhibiting neuronal activity.

The GABA receptor contains distinct binding sites for several CNS drugs, including anxiolytics, anticonvulsants, and sedative hypnotics. Whilst GABA binds to a site at the interface of alpha and beta subunits, most CNS drugs acting at the receptor interact through allosteric sites elsewhere on the receptor. The most extensively studied of these drugs are the benzodiazepines; as mentioned previously, these drugs were discovered in the clinic and their site of action was determined through reverse pharmacology. Although the initial benzodiazepine drugs such as diazepam are highly effective anxiolytics, their use is limited by significant side-effects including sedation, cognitive impairment, and tolerance/ withdrawal. These effects are all most likely mediated through interactions with $GABA_A$ receptors; however, it is clear that anxiolytic and sedative effects are mediated by receptors consisting of different combinations of specific subunits. Thus mice engineered to have an inactive α1 subunit are resistant to the sedative effects of benzodiazepines, but retain the anxiolytic-like effects. Conversely mice engineered to have inactive α2 subunits do not demonstrate the anxiolytic-like effects of benzodiazepines but do demonstrate sedation. Based on these observations, a number of drug discovery efforts have focused on generating subtype-selected $GABA_A$ receptor modulators. It is proven to be possible to develop subtype-preferring agents as sedative/hypnotics, although these compounds are not truly selective.

More recent approaches have moved away from the benzodiazepine structure into related structures with improved selectivity potential; currently approved drugs include zolpidem and eszopiclone, both of which preferentially target the α1-containing receptors.

It has proven considerably more difficult to target α2 receptors selectively. Several compounds have been described which are α2/α3-preferring partial agonists, with potential as novel anxiolytic drugs. Whilst these compounds have been shown to have a nonsedating, anxiolytic-like action in animal models, it is not yet clear whether this translates to an anxiolytic effect in patients. Attempts at refining this approach are hampered by two factors; firstly the difficulty in understanding how studies in transgenic mice on the role of different receptor subunits translates to man in terms of both subunit composition and anatomical distribution. Given the complexity of receptor composition, it is quite possible that other subunits are involved in the anxiolytic effects in man. Secondly, whilst it has been possible to retain $GABA_A$ receptor modulation in structures other than benzodiazepines, it has not been possible to devise robust and reliable screening assays suitable for use with diverse chemical libraries, and it has been difficult to identify novel structures with greater potential for selective interactions.

Secretases and Alzheimer's disease

An interesting example of the use of novel fragment-based approaches to lead generation is provided by β-secretase (Edwards *et al.*, 2007). β-Secretase is a membrane-bound aspartyl protease responsible for the cleavage of the amyloid precursor protein to produce the γ-secretase substrate C99 (Figure 4) and as such is a highly attractive target for novel disease-modifying approaches to Alzheimer's disease. β-Secretase is unusual in that it is the first example of a pepsin family aspartyl transferase which occurs as a transmembrane protein. Initially substrate analog peptidic inhibitors of β-secretase were described with high potency and selectivity. Attempts to produce more drug-like inhibitors based on a peptidomimetic approach have not been successful. Similarly the identification of small molecule inhibitors with good drug-like properties from high-throughput screening has also been difficult. The crystal structure of β-secretase has been determined, and it appears that the substrate binding pocket of the enzyme is distinct from other pepsin-like proteases and contains a large, poorly defined binding pocket for the natural substrate. The crystal structure has been successfully incorporated in more recent approaches based on low-affinity fragment binding. In one such study, low-affinity binding of low molecular weight fragments was identified using NMR-based techniques. Crystallographic analysis of these fragments bound to β-secretase identified a novel interaction with the aspartyl residues at the active site, and led to the development of novel series of drug-like inhibitors (Edwards *et al.*, 2007).

Optimizing small molecules as CNS drug candidates

It is not the purpose of this review to cover all aspects of lead optimization. There are, however, several aspects which are particularly relevant to CNS therapeutics. Most prominent amongst these is the challenge of drug delivery to the CNS, overcoming both systemic and brain barriers to achieve robust and reliable drug exposure at the target site. The major obstacle to drug delivery to the CNS is the blood-brain barrier, a consequence of the unique structure of brain capillaries which limits the uptake of compounds and extrudes compounds which are present in the brain. Brain capillaries are encased by vascular endothelial cells which are connected through tight junctions maintained by specific cell adhesion molecules. In addition, astrocytic projections surround the endo-thelial cells, thus providing a physical barrier to the passage of large molecules into the brain extracellular fluid. Several in vitro models of the blood-brain barrier have been described, and together with in vivo analysis of transport into the brain these systems have provided much information on the optimal properties of compounds which correlate with good CNS uptake. Lipophilicity has long been known to influence CNS drug uptake, supporting passive permeability across neuronal membranes. The presence of ionizable groups is another major factor, with permeation of the ionized species generally at least 1000-fold lower. In addition, ampipathic cations are also accumulated in the brain depending upon membrane potential and pH trapping. Other factors with major effects include the number of hydrogen bonding groups, molecular weight, and polar surface area of molecules (Lipinski *et al.*, 1997).

As if this is not enough, further complication is added by the presence of an array of transporters mediating efflux from the CNS, including P-glycoprotein (PGP) and the MRP family of transporters (Liu *et al.*, 2008). PGP is an ATP-dependent efflux pump found in many endothelial cells, but particularly in the brain. The MRP transporters, of which at least six are involved in drug transport, are also present in brain endothelial cells and act as ATP-dependent efflux pumps. The substrate specificity of PGP and MRP is broad, and the lack of specificity makes it extremely difficult to generate structure activity predictions. Although some in silico models exist, screening lead compounds through transporter assays and blood-brain barrier models has become an essential, integral part of CNS drug optimization. In addition to the above factors, for many drugs the free plasma concentration is the main determinant of brain entry. Plasma free concentrations depend in turn on the rate of absorption and entry into the systemic circulation, and on the degree of plasma protein binding. These factors bring an additional set of physicochemical and structural constraints for optimization of lead compounds. In many cases optimization to ensure good brain exposure requires balancing a set of structural requirements which also enhance the possibility of increasing affinity for drug-metabolizing enzymes and increasing affinity for cardiac ion channels.

Based on the above considerations, it can be seen that optimizing these properties (loosely referred to as drug-like properties) whilst maintaining all of the other properties generally required of a viable drug candidate is a complex, unpredictable process requiring many iterative steps of chemical modification, followed by testing of physicochemical and biological properties and design of new molecules based on the obtained data (see Gabrielsson *et al.*, 2009, for discussion).

Biologics as CNS drugs

In the early 1980s the pharmaceutical industry was revolutionized by the first recombinant protein therapeutic (human insulin) entering the market. Since that time, multiple technology platforms for the development of therapeutics using recombinant proteins and monoclonal antibodies (MAbs) have been developed to treat a variety of diseases. Biopharmaceuticals are predominantly protein-based molecules that can function as agonists, antagonists, or as replacement for a missing or malfunctioning protein. Biologic drugs offer two attractive advantages over small molecules as potential CNS agents. Firstly, selectivity, which is often a problem with small molecules, is usually extremely good. Secondly, many targets which have not proven amenable to small molecule interaction such as protein-protein interactions can be addressed with biologics. However, whilst many biopharmaceuticals have become extremely successful drugs for the treatment of a wide variety of illnesses, only a few have found utility in CNS disorders. There are a number of major hurdles to be addressed with regard to biologics in CNS therapeutics, the most challenging being overcoming the blood-brain barrier, which under normal circumstances is impermeable to proteins and nucleic acids. The practical issues of route of drug administration (i.e. use of injectables) and the high cost of biologics relative to the cost of small molecule treatments are major drawbacks. However, new technologies in blood-brain barrier penetration and administration devices and lowering cost of goods are addressing all of these issues.

Currently two classes of biologics have been launched for the CNS (Pavlou and Reichert, 2004):

- Thrombolytics for the acute treatment of stroke. The basic mechanism of action of thrombolytic agents is the activation of plasminogen to form plasmin and in turn mediate cleavage of fibrin, the major component of the blood clot. This approach was based on treatment strategy in acute myocardial infarction where the efficacy of streptokinase has been established for many years. However, the great sensitivity of the brain to the hemorrhagic effects of streptokinase prevented its use in stroke treatment. Tissue plasminogen activator (tPA) is associated with considerably lower risk of hemorrhage and is the most commonly used agent. A number of recombinant tPAs are available; of these only Alteplase is approved for the treatment of acute ischemic stroke. r-tPA is administered intravenously to ischemic stroke patients within 3 hours of symptom onset; some studies suggest that direct arterial administration of r-tPA is more effective in certain types of stroke.
- Biologics in the treatment of multiple sclerosis. Three interferon β recombinant proteins have been approved for the treatment of MS. The mechanism of action of these proteins is unknown, but it is generally inferred to involve modulation of the pathogenic immune process.

In these cases, the active biologic agent is a recombinant human protein with no further modification. Although these are viable treatment options bringing benefit to many patients, a number of drawbacks are documented. The stability and plasma half-life may not be optimal, and in some cases the production of neutralizing antibodies can be an issue. Moreover, the cost of such treatments can be high and calculations of cost benefit can be unfavorable. Such considerations act as powerful drivers for the modification of biologics to optimize these parameters.

Pre-clinical development of CNS biologics

Pre-clinical development of biologics starts with a screening process analogous to the high-throughput screening used for small molecules (Brekke and Sandlie, 2003). In the case of monoclonal antibodies, libraries containing several millions of antibody fragments can be used to assess in vitro target binding. These libraries can be screened at a rate of more than 1000 clones per day in cell-based assays. Typically between 5000 and 50 000 clones will be screened for any one campaign. Like their small molecule counterparts, biotherapeutics are also optimized to enhance the affinity and specificity of the agent for its biological target, to modify the mechanism of interaction, or to alter the in vivo uptake or clearance of the molecule. The affinity of an antibody can be increased by engineering the specific regions using technologies such as phage or ribosome display. If the lead antibody is rodent in origin it can be humanized by grafting specific portions of the rodent antibody onto human constant domains, thus rendering the antibody less immunogenic to man. Additionally, proteins are optimized for maximum expression in cellular systems, maximum product quality, homogeneity, stability, and solubility. Further changes can be made to enhance biological stability and the inclusion of additional functional domains. More recently, in addition to protein-based biologics, biopharmaceuticals are extending to nucleic acid-based or other novel technologies such as RNA interference (RNAi) and aptamers.

Translational neuroscience and pre-clinical development

Translational research is defined as "the transfer of knowledge gained from basic research to new and improved methods of preventing, diagnosing, or treating disease, as well as the transfer of clinical insights into hypotheses that can be tested and validated in the basic research laboratory" (Hall, 2002). The goal is to provide a better understanding of the disease in question by linking basic and clinical research at every stage of the drug R&D value chain. Driven totally by data, it is a two-way iterative process where drug discovery and development is complemented by the pursuit of understanding human diseases. In forward translation, one will use pre-clinical findings to guide clinical studies and the development plan (e.g. disease indications, patient populations, dose selection, dosing regimen). In back-translation, one will use clinical data to improve pre-clinical drug discovery (e.g. identify and validate drug targets, understand disease mechanisms, develop predictive models/biomarkers).

Animal models used in most drug discovery efforts do not mimic the human diseases in question. In no other therapeutic area is this more relevant than diseases of the CNS. Therefore significant risk is taken when compounds are brought to clinic trials without reassuring data that the mechanism in question has disease relevance. This risk can be reduced, however, through rigorous scientific validation of the target. Further, there needs to be assurance that the target in question has interacted with the molecule in the appropriate fashion (agonist, antagonist, inhibition, modulation), eliciting a measurable pharmacodynamic response. Translational research involving proof of mechanism (POM), proof of concept (POC), and proof of safety (POS) studies based on biomarker analysis is critical for yielding early information to make crucial decisions on the probability of clinical success of a new chemical entity.

Biomarkers in CNS therapies

Quality biomarkers demonstrate sensitivity, can be measured easily, and correlate with disease activity. Minimally, biomarkers will aid in measuring the response to a therapeutic intervention (Biomarkers Definition Working Group, 2001). Based on the information they reveal, biomarkers for CNS disorders can be classified as biochemical, neuroimaging, clinical (endophenotyping), and pharmacogenetic.

Identifying biochemical biomarkers in blood and CSF for CNS disorders has predominantly focused on the assaying of single metabolites. This has not been a fruitful area of translational information based on the central nature of the disorder, specifically dealing with blood brain issues. Often hypothesis-driven, there has not been significant success demonstrated through this approach. Often the biomarkers in question do not have the desired sensitivity and specificity for use in diagnosis or serve as surrogate endpoints in clinical trials for drug efficacy, nor have sufficient power to identify disorders at an early stage (Quinones and Kaddurah-Daouk, 2009). As an example, the measurement of multiple biochemical analytes in blood, urine, and cerebrospinal fluid such as β-amyloid or tau proteins has been proposed in Alzheimer's disease due to their involvement in the pathophysiology of the disease (Sunderland *et al.*, 2003). However, when measured, none of these biomarkers is linearly related to the stage of the disease (Gurwitz, 2002). Further, with several different therapeutic approaches advancing which are predicated on different aspects of disease pathophysiology, measurement of biomarkers other than those that are amyloid or tau-based may be required (Frank and Hargreaves, 2003).

Neuroimaging biomarkers emanate from state-of-the-art imaging technologies such as positron emission tomography (PET) and single photon emission computerized tomography (SPECT) used for measuring the labeling and displacement of isotope-labeled ligands for receptors, soluble enzymes, and ion channels. Further, magnetic resonance (MRI) and functional magnetic resonance imaging (fMRI) yield high resolution of activity in specific brain regions which makes this a potentially useful translational tool. These methods involve the measurement of region-specific changes in the oxygen content of the blood in microcirculation which provides an indirect measurement in cerebral blood flow and neural activity. Neuroimaging techniques, when used in combination with one another, can be powerful translational tools not only for assessing CNS disorders but also in establishing the PK/PD relationship, which is a cornerstone to driving effective drug development with accurate dose-ranging studies (Borsook *et al.*, 2006). Biomarker measurements from these techniques which supplement clinical data are being used in a variety of CNS disorders including Parkinson's disease (Berg, 2008), Alzheimer's disease (Jagust, 2004), bipolar disorder (Phillips and Vieta, 2007), and Huntington's disease (Rosas *et al.*, 2004). With any method, there are strengths and weaknesses to the approach. Clearly, measurement of these biomarkers provides important diagnostic and predictive drug treatment information and can be performed repeatedly at any stage of the disease process. Costs, the limitations of how and where patients can be tested, and exposure to radioactive probes can be concerns when using these techniques.

Clinically standard techniques which have now come into vogue for generating translational data in pre-clinical and clinical studies are electrophysiology and electroencephalography (EEG). This technique is currently being utilized as a non-invasive translational pharmacodynamic marker in the CNS. Scalp recorded magnetoencephalography (MEG) and event-related potentials (ERPs) can also provide measures of brain electrical activity in healthy volunteers and patients. Moreover, several specific electrophysiological measures are pre-attentional (e.g. P50, mismatch negativity) and do not require attentional or purposeful actions of the test subject (Naatanen and Kahkonen, 2009). There is a clear advantage offered over neuropsychological evaluations, which affect an individual's vigilance and motivational state. There is a strong face validity and mechanistic homology across rodents, primates, and humans for a battery of EEG/ERP components, supporting valuable pre-clinical to clinical translation. An example is the cross-species measurement of schizophrenia-related sensorimotor gating deficit using pre-pulse inhibition (PPI) of startle paradigm (Light and Braff, 1999; Swerdlow *et al.*, 2008).

There is increased use of objective translational tools to define relevant endophenotypes/intermediate phenotypes, which can be used in certain clinical settings to aid in the identification of genetic heterogeneity within a given disease population. An endophenotype is a biological or behavioral feature (in non-affected subjects or patients) that reflects a discrete biological system, and as such is thought to be more closely related to a specific gene than the broad clinical phenotype (Insel and Cuthbert, 2009). It is expected to augment the discriminating power of genetic association and linkage studies, as well as facilitating the development of new therapeutics targeting subsets of complex phenotypes (Gottesman and Gould, 2003; Meyer-Lindenberg and Weinberger, 2006; Tan *et al.*, 2008). An example of an endophenotype is deficient sensorimotor gating, i.e. a reduction in the brain's ability to filter excessive sensory information and generate appropriate motor responses as measured by prepulse inhibition (PPI). PPI deficits can be seen in schizophrenia as well as bipolar disorder (Giakoumaki *et al.*, 2007). Indeed, substantial genetic overlap has been reported for schizophrenia and bipolar disorders (Le-Niculescu *et al.*, 2007). Since PPI can be measured in rodents and primates it can be used translationally across pre-clinical and clinical studies to identify and confirm drug candidates in these various disease domains.

Using pharmacogenetic/pharmacogenomic biomarkers for aiding drug discovery, development, and patient segmentation in a variety of different CNS diseases should be considered an emerging technology. Utilizing this approach, treatments can be designed for specific individuals through information gained on the genetics of disease and drug mechanism and will serve as the basis for the future of personalized healthcare. Currently, clinically significant polymorphisms are being used to not only identify patients at risk of developing certain diseases, but also help identify patients most likely to gain benefit with specific therapies through either greater efficacy or reduced incidence of side effects. Genotypes (single nucleotide polymorphisms, SNPs) and haplotypes can serve as biomarkers for clinical phenotypes. As an example, the primary target of selective serotonin reuptake inhibitors (SSRIs) is the serotonin transporter, and the inter-individual variation in clinical response to an SSRI may be related to inter-subject variability in 5-HT transporter (5-HTT) expression (Spigset and Martensson, 1999).

A common polymorphism in the human 5-HTT gene (SLC6A4) resulting in the short (s) and long (l) variants in the promoter region of the gene has been studied extensively. This polymorphism impacts the 5-HTT gene transcriptional efficiency and expression in transfected cells, the s allele associated with lower transcription, expression, and activity of the 5-HTT (Mancama and Kerwin, 2003). Interestingly, individuals homozygous for the s allele are associated with heightened anxiety and more readily develop affective illness than the l allele carriers (Lesch and Mossner, 1998). Further, several clinical studies in depressed patients have reported differences in the efficacy and time of onset of SSRIs associated with variations in this 5-HTT LPR polymorphism and those with the l/l genotype have a more favorable and earlier-onset response to SSRI treatments than the s allele carriers, although there are also some conflicting data (Kato *et al.*, 2005; Luddington *et al.*, 2009). It should be noted, however, that most CNS diseases result from complex gene interactions and environmental factors (Kiberstis and Roberts, 2002). Therefore genetic predisposition only provides information about relative risk as the disease expression is influenced by other factors.

The development of new biomarkers is critical to the clinical success of new chemical entities targeting newly validated targets for a variety of CNS diseases. Biomarkers are critical to managing the inherent risk in CNS drug discovery and development and those programs which contain a lucid translational strategy should be given priority. Having a strong cadre of biomarkers in a CNS discovery/development effort allows for strong cost-containment and simpler decision-making and helps get new therapeutics to the right patient population faster.

Conclusions and future prospects

Considerable advances have been made in understanding the basic neurobiology and pathophysiology of many neuropsychiatric disorders. Novel targets for disease modification in Alzheimer's disease are in clinical development and other targets in the amyloid pathway are at earlier stages of development. In this case, advances derived from genetic studies and molecular neurobiology have been critical to identifying and advancing these targets. Targets relating to glutamatergic mechanisms are generating interesting clinical data in the treatment of severe depression and possibly schizophrenia. It has been advances in genomics, molecular pharmacology, and functional imaging which have driven interest in these targets. It is interesting to note that in both cases new targets and understanding of disease mechanisms are derived from a broad range of neuroscience advances and technological innovation, but still rely on back-translation from the clinic. These advances have not been limited to the major neuropsychiatric illnesses currently treated with large "blockbuster" drugs. For example, considerable interest has been generated in the treatment of fragile X syndrome with metabotropic glutamate receptor antagonists and new novel targets are emerging for a variety of currently untreated orphan CNS illnesses.

It is of course not new seeing several encouraging, novel therapies in clinical development for neuropsychiatric disorders; unfortunately in the past very few of these have actually delivered their promise. It is well documented that many of these disappointments are due to failure to engage the drug target appropriately in the right patient population, or the fact that the choice of target is wrong. It is a reasonable expectation that advances in drug discovery and implementation of translational approaches will increase our ability to ensure effective target engagement. The increased understanding of disease mechanisms permits the development of models based on integrative physiological and pharmacological approaches, in contrast to a predominantly black box approach used in the past.

Whilst these advances have been promising, much remains to be done to ensure a continuous flow of relevant drug targets into the drug discovery process. As discussed, this in turn relies on increased understanding of disease biology and the translation of this knowledge into disease models capable of supporting rigorous validation and translation, in turn increasing the confidence of efficacy in the clinic. As new targets are taken to proof concept in the clinic, the underlying disease model or hypothesis is critically tested, thus building confidence in the model through an iterative process.

Our ability to perform definitive clinical efficacy experiments necessary to test the validation of novel targets is critical to this process. It is noteworthy that whilst proof of clinical efficacy is invaluable in this iterative process of hypothesis testing, efficacy alone may not be sufficient to support the costly investment in drug development post pre-clinical research. With regard to the diseases with established treatments which are only partially effective, new treatments need to provide improved efficacy or provide efficacy in patient subgroups in which current treatments are ineffective. In terms of disease models and mechanisms, understanding the action of current treatments and the role of their targets is essential to identifying targets with potential for improved therapies.

It is clear from this discussion that an effective interface between basic research into disease mechanisms and the identification and validation of targets of interest to pre-clinical drug development is one of the key challenges. In this regard one can view the interaction between academic and government-funded basic research and biotech/ pharma drug discovery as one of mutual interdependence and potential synergy. This interdependence stretches beyond the mutual interaction at the pre-clinical stage to equally important interdependencies at the translational and clinical development phases, which are outside the scope of this chapter. A number of important precompetitive consortia have emerged to bridge the industry-academia interface at this early phase of drug discovery, with the intention of facilitating the advances in disease biology and sharing the risks in bringing novel approaches into the development process.

These interactions in precompetitive research are essential to the future of CNS drug discovery and it is to be hoped that such interactions will bring innovative impactful treatments addressing the enormous unmet needs in these debilitating disorders.

References

Agid, Y., Buzsáki, G., and Diamond, D. M. (2007). How can drug discovery for psychiatric disorders be improved? *Nat Rev Drug Discov*, 6, 189–201.

Arguello, P. A. and Gogos, J. A. (2006). Modeling madness in mice: one piece at a time. *Neuron*, 52, 179–96.

Atkinson, A. J., Jr., Colburn, W. A., DeGruttola, V. G., et al. (2001). *Clin Pharmacol Thera*, 69, 89–95.

Babaoglu, K. and Shiochet, B. K. (2006). Deconstructing fragment based inhibitor discovery. *Nat Chem Biol*, 2, 720–33.

Berg, D. (2008). Biomarkers for the early detection of Parkinson's and Alzheimer's Disease. *Neurodegen Dis*, 5, 133–6.

Borsook, D., Bacerra, L., and Hargreaves, R. (2006). A role for fMRI in optimizing CNS drug development. *Nat Rev Drug Discov*, 5, 411–425.

Brekke, O. H. and Sandlie, I. (2003). Therapeutic antibodies for human diseases at the dawn of the twenty-first century. *Nat Rev Drug Discov*, 2, 52–62.

Cheng, A. C., Coleman, R. G., Smyth, K. T., et al. (2007). Structure-based maximal affinity model predicts small-molecule druggability. *Nat Biotechnol*, 25, 71–75.

Chico, L. K., Van Eldik, L. J., and Watterson, D. M. (2009). Targeting protein kinases in central nervous system disorders. *Nat Rev Drug Discov*, 8, 893–909.

Citron, M. (2010). Alzheimer's disease: strategies for disease modification. *Nat Rev Drug Discov*, 9, 387–98.

Edwards, P. D., Albert, J. S., Sylvester, M., et al. (2007). Application of fragment based lead generation to the discovery of novel cyclic amidine b-secretase inhibitors with nanomolar potency, cellular activity and high ligand efficiency. *J Med Chem*, 50, 5912–25.

Frank, R. and Hargreaves, R. (2003). Clinical markers in drug discovery and development. *Nat Rev Drug Discov*, 2, 566–80.

Gabrielsson, J., Dolgos, H., Gillberg, P.-G., et al. (2009). Early integration of pharmacokinetic and dynamic reasoning is essential for optimal development of lead compounds: strategic considerations. *Drug Discov Today*, 14, 358–72.

Giakoumaki, S. G., Roussos, P., Rogdaki, M., et al. (2007). Evidence of disrupted prepulse inhibition in unaffected siblings of bipolar disorder patients. *Biol Psychiat*, 62, 1418–22.

Gottesman, I. I. and Gould, T.D. (2003). The endophenotype concept in psychiatry: etymology and strategic intentions. *Am J Psychiat*, 160, 636–45.

Gould, T. G. and Gottesman, I. I. (2006). Psychiatric endophenotypes and the development of valid animal models. *Gene Brain Behav*, 5, 113–19.

Gurwitz, D. (2002). Targeting Alzheimer's disease: is there a light at the end of the tunnel? *Drug Dev Res*, 56, 45–8.

Hall, J. E. (2002). The promise of translational physiology. *Am J Physiol*, L235–6.

Heilker, R., Wolff, M., Tautermann, C. S., et al. (2009). G-protein coupled receptor-focused drug discovery using a target class platform approach. *Drug Discov Today*, 5/6, 231–44.

Imming, P., Sinning, C., and Meyer, A. (2006). Drugs, their targets and the nature and number of drug targets. *Nat Rev Drug Discov*, 5, 821–34.

Insel, T. R. and Cuthbert, B. N. (2009). Endophenotypes: bridging genomic complexity and disorder heterogeneity, *Biol Psychiatry*, 66 (11), 988–9.

Jagust, W. (2004). Molecular neuroimaging in Alzheimer's disease. *NeuroRX*, 1, 206–12.

Jorgensen, W. L. (2009). Efficient drug lead discovery and optimization. *Accounts Chem Res*, 42, 724–33.

Kato, M., Ikenaga, Y., Wakeno, M., *et al.* (2005). Controlled clinical comparison of paroxetine and fluvoxamine considering the serotonin transporter promoter polymorphism. *Int Clin Psychopharmacol*, 20, 151–6.

Kiberstis, P. and Roberts, L. (2002). It's not just the genes. *Science*, 296, 685.

Knowles, J. and Gromo, G. (2003). Target selection in drug discovery. *Nat Rev Drug Discov*, 2, 63–9.

Krishnamurthy, H., Piscitelli, C. L., and Gouaux, E. (2009). Unlocking the molecular secrets of sodium-coupled transporters. *Nature*, 459, 347–55.

Le-Niculescu, H., Balaraman, Y., Patel, S., *et al.* (2007). Towards understanding the schizophrenia code: an expanded convergent functional genomics approach. *Am J Med Genet, Neuropsychiatr Genet*, 144B, 129–58.

Lesch, K. P. and Mossner, R. (1998). Genetically driven variation in serotonin uptake: is there a link to affective spectrum, neurodevelopmental, and neurodegenerative disorders? *Biol Psychiatry*, 44, 179–92.

Light, G. A. and Braff, D. L. (1999). Human and animal studies of schizophrenia related gating deficits. *Curr Psychiatr Rep*, 1, 31–40.

Lindsay, M. A. (2003). Target discovery. *Nat Rev Drug Discov*, 2, 831–8.

Lipinski, C., Lombardo, F., Dominy, B., *et al.* (1997). Experimental and computational approaches to estimate solubility and permeability in drug discovery and development settings. *Adv Drug Deliver Rev*, 23, 3–25.

Liu, X., Chen, C., and Smith, B. J. (2008). Progress in brain penetration evaluation in drug discovery and development. *J Pharmacol Exp Ther*, 325, 349–56.

Luddington, N. S., Mandadapu, A., Husk, M., *et al.* (2009). Clinical implications of genetic variation in the serotonin transporter promoter region: a review. *Primary Care Companion J Clin Psychiatr*, 11, 93–102.

Mancama, D. and Kerwin, R. W. (2003). Role of pharmacogenetics in individualising treatment with SSRIs. *CNS Drugs*, 17, 1–10.

Meyer-Lindenberg, A. and Weinberger, D. (2006). Intermediate phenotypes and genetic mechanisms of psychiatric disorders. *Nat Rev Neurosci*, 7, 818–27.

Naatanen, R. and Kahkonen, S. (2009). Central auditory dysfunction in schizophrenia as revealed by the mismatch negativity (MMN) and its magnetic equivalent MMNm: a review. *Int J Neuropsychopharmacol*, 12, 125–35.

Overington, J. P., Al-Lazikani, B., and Hopkins, A. L. (2006). How many drug targets are there? *Nat Rev Drug Discov*, 5, 993–1002.

Pangalos, M. N., Schechter, L. E., and Hurko, O. (2007). Drug development for CNS disorders: strategies for balancing risk and reducing attrition. *Nat Rev Drug Discov*, 6, 521–32.

Paolini, G. V., Shapland, R. H. B., van Hoorn, W. P., *et al.* (2006). Global mapping of pharmacological space. *Nat Biotechnol*, 24, 805–15.

Pavlou, A. K. and Reichert, J. M. (2004). Recombinant protein therapeutics success rates, market trends and values to 2010. *Nat Biotechnol*, 22, 1513–19.

Philipson, O., Lord, A., Gumucio, A., *et al.* (2010). Animal models of amyloid-b-related pathologies in Alzheimers disease. *FEBS J*, 277, 1389–409.

Phillips, M. L. and Vieta, E. (2007). Identifying functional neuroimaging biomarkers of bipolar disorders: Towards DSM-V. *Schizophrenia Bull*, 33, 893–904.

Quinones, M. P. and Kaddurah-Daouk, R. (2009). Metabolomics tools for identifying biomarkers for neuropsychiatric diseases. *Neurobiol Dis*, 35, 165–176.

Rosas, H. D., Feigin, H. S., and Hersch, S. M. (2004). Using advances in neuroimaging to detect, understand, and monitor disease progression in Huntington's disease. *NeuroRX*, 1, 263–272.

Sarter, M. (2006). Preclinical research into cognition enhancers. *Trends Pharmacol Sci*, 27, 602–8.

Schmidtke, P. and Barril, X. (2010). Understanding and predicting druggability. A high-throughput method for detection of drug binding sites. *J Med Chem*, 53, 5858–67.

Spedding, M., Jay, T., Costa, J., *et al.* (2005). A pathophysiological paradigm for the therapy of psychiatric disease. *Nat Rev Drug Discov*, 4, 467–76.

Spigset, O. and Martensson, B. (1999). Fortnightly review: drug treatment of depression. *Brit Med J*, 318, 1188–91.

Sunderland, T., Linker, G., Nadeem, M., *et al.* (2003). Decreased β-amyloid 1–42 and increased Tau levels in cerebrospinal fluid of patients with Alzheimer's disease. *J Am Med Assoc*, 289, 2094–103.

Swerdlow, N. R., Weber, M., Qu, Y., *et al.* (2008). Realistic expectations of prepulse inhibition in translational models for schizophrenia research. *Psychopharmacology*, 199, 331–88.

Tan, H. Y., Callicott, J. H., and Weinberger, D. R. (2008). Intermediate phenotypes in schizophrenia genetics redux: is it a no brainer? *Mol Psychiatry*, 13, 233–8.

Whiting, P. (2003). GABA-A receptor subtypes in the brain: a paradigm for drug discovery? *Drug Discov Today*, 8, 445–52.

Wu, G. and Doberstein, S. K. (2006). HTS technologies in biopharmaceutical discovery. *Drug Discov Today*, 11, 718–26.

Wulff, H., Castle, N. A., and Pardo, L. A. (2009). Voltage-gated potassium channels as therapeutic targets. *Nat Rev Drug Discov*, 8, 98–1001.

Zimmermann, G. R., Lehar, J., and Keith, C. T. (2007). Multi-target therapeutics: when the whole is greater than the sum of the parts. *Drug Discov Today*, 12, 34–42.

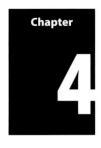

Phase I trials: from traditional to newer approaches

Matthew Macaluso, Michael Krams, and
Sheldon Preskorn

Introduction

Phase I clinical trials have traditionally been focused on populations of normal healthy volunteers with the goal of determining the safety, tolerability, and pharmacokinetic profile of new investigational agents. As CNS drug development shifts its focus to the development of novel molecular entities, this approach will undergo an evolution.

Phase I studies are traditionally focused on determining the safety, tolerability, and pharmacokinetics of a new molecular entity in young healthy volunteers – first in a single ascending dose (SAD) study and then in a multiple ascending dose (MAD) study (Spilker, 1991). The goal of this chapter is to help clinicians and researchers better understand the strengths and weaknesses of this classic approach. We first review the rationale for and design of Phase I studies. We then discuss how Phase I studies are expanding to examine the effects of drugs in specific target populations, exploring both traditional endpoints and newer biomarker endpoints selected specifically to test the potential utility of the drug on the target illness (Wong *et al.*, 2009). We will focus especially on the expansion of Phase I studies to gather data in a time- and cost-effective fashion that will allow sponsors to determine whether or not to proceed ("go/no-go") with a new investigational molecule (Gallo *et al.*, 2006). The second half will discuss how the development of novel molecular entities (NMEs) designed specifically to affect the central nervous system (CNS) creates challenges that cannot be addressed solely by the traditional approach, which will need to be augmented by new methodological strategies (Paul *et al.*, 2010).

Traditional early-phase design considerations

The authors subscribe to Sheiner's proposal to distinguish between the "learn" and "confirm" phases of drug development (Sheiner, 1997). In the "learn" phase (Phases I and II, exploratory clinical development), the goal is first to establish whether the NME is safe and well tolerated and has an appropriate pharmacokinetic (PK) profile and then to move on to the initial proof of concept efficacy trials. At its simplest level, the traditional Phase I development of an NME consists of one initial SAD study followed by one MAD study in normal volunteers.

Traditionally, the first step in Phase I development is a single dose administration of the NME. These studies typically involve six to nine subjects who receive the NME and two to three additional subjects who receive placebo, with assignments to the groups made in a

Essential CNS Drug Development, ed. A. Kalali, Sheldon Preskorn, J. Kwentus, and Stephen M. Stahl. Published by Cambridge University Press. © Cambridge University Press 2012.

double-blind, randomized manner. This approach permits the investigators to document differences in serious or nuisance adverse effects that occur with high frequency (i.e. in more than 1 in 4 patients). After each dose level is administered, safety and tolerability are assessed before determining whether to administer a higher dose and if so, how much higher. The goal of these studies is to establish the maximum tolerated single dose (MTD) of the NME (McConnell, 1989). The design typically includes clearly laid out decision rules on whether or not to escalate to the next dose level, given the observations at previous dose levels (Dragalin, 2006).

Key questions involved in the design of a traditional SAD study include:

- What is the starting dose? The initial dose chosen for the SAD study is typically below the no observable effect level (NOEL) in animals (Crane and Newman, 2000).
- What is the escalation scheme (i.e. what multiple of the last dose is used for the next dose)?
- What constitutes a dose-limiting safety or tolerability problem, given the indication that is ultimately being sought?

The goal is to learn about the following (Arbuck, 1996):

- Are the pharmacokinetics (PK) of the compound suitable for use as a clinical agent, including time to peak concentration (T_{max}), peak concentration (C_{max}), half-life ($T_{1/2}$), trough concentration (C_{min}), and dose-drug concentration linearity over the dose range studied?
- Are the PK of the molecule related to its pharmacodynamics (PD), including onset of effect (T_{max}), duration of effect ($T_{1/2}$), and intensity of effect (C_{max} and C_{min})?
- What is the nature of the drug's PD in terms of both desired and undesired effects?
- What dose should be chosen based on the SAD results and knowledge from preclinical models to take into the MAD study?

At the end of an SAD study, the following should ideally have been determined:

- The MTD and
- PK/PD relationship for safety and tolerability.

However, a number of important learning points may not be achieved by the simplest traditional SAD study, such as:

- Does the NME – assuming it is being developed for a CNS indication – penetrate into the brain?
- Does the NME achieve a concentration at its intended site of action that is likely to produce a therapeutic effect?
- Does the NME have an effect on a biomarker that should be predictive of efficacy in the therapeutic indication for which it is being developed?

All of these points can be studied in normal volunteers but they may also need to be studied in patients with the target illness, either to assess for the desired effect or because the dose-response curve may shift in the population with the target illness compared to normal volunteers. In such cases, it may be worth planning the study so that one or more cohorts of subjects who approximate the target populations can be studied after the initial studies are done in normal volunteers (i.e. a seamless transition from normal to symptomatic volunteers). An example of this would be the development

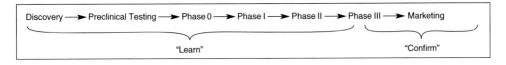

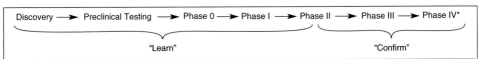

Figure 1. "Learn and confirm" phases of drug development.

of an NME for dementia of the Alzheimer's type. This could involve a multi-step process, going from healthy young volunteers to healthy elderly volunteers to elderly volunteers with a mild form of the target illness. Since Alzheimer's dementia occurs predominantly in elderly patients, it is important to determine if the safety, tolerability, and even the PK of the NME differ between young healthy volunteers and elderly healthy volunteers.

After completing an SAD study, an MAD study is conducted to better understand the PK and PD of multiple doses of the NME. The designs and goals of the SAD and MAD studies are generally the same, except that, in the MAD study, the drug is administered to the volunteers for one or more weeks on a daily basis, or even multiple times per day depending on the drug's half-life as determined in the SAD study. The initial doses for this study are based on the SAD study and are generally higher than the starting doses used in the SAD study but almost always lower than the MTD determined in the SAD study. Otherwise, the design is comparable in terms of number of subjects receiving the NME versus placebo, and the dose escalation is again based on the results of the previous dosing group. Again, the MAD study may be designed to transition into the age range for the target population and/or into a mildly affected group having the target illness.

The distinction between late Phase I and early Phase II studies may not always be clearly demarcated, and a study may straddle the boundary between traditional Phase I and early Phase II. Thus, the participants in the early groups in an SAD and/or MAD study are traditionally young healthy volunteers, whereas later volunteers may have the target illness. The goal of including these latter cohorts in these studies may be to provide an early test of mechanism and/or concept to determine whether the NME has the properties required to have a reasonable chance of success in Phase III studies (see Figure 1). In the "confirm" phase (i.e. Phase III), the goal is to produce substantial evidence that a treatment regimen applied to a particular patient population achieves a specific endpoint that is accepted by regulatory agencies as being efficacious and will yield a sufficient effect size relative to any safety or tolerability concerns to warrant approval (Kraemer *et al.*, 2003). "Confirm" is about hypothesis testing, and the main customers are regulatory agencies (Sheiner, 1997). However, throughout the process, principally before entering Phase III testing, the goal is to efficiently identify viable and non-viable compounds and focus resources on the former and discontinue further development of the latter.

CNS drug development is facing challenges that will drastically affect the way both parts of the "learn" and "confirm" dichotomy will be conducted (Paul *et al.*, 2010). Essentially, psychiatric drug development has mainly been "living off" chlorpromazine and its derivatives for 50 years and now has entered the era of the human genome project, which is producing more targets than large Pharma can afford to pursue efficiently. Hence, CNS drug development must "evolve", to be more efficient in making "go/no-go" decisions.

How Phase I studies are being challenged

To understand the future, one must be cognizant of the past. A review of the last 30 years of CNS drug development reveals that CNS clinical trial designs have been largely static (Kaitin, 2010). Over this period, this approach has made sense because newer drugs were by and large a molecular refinement of previous molecules, with minor although sometimes clinically important changes in either PD or PK. However, the process of refining chlorpromazine and its derivatives appears to have been virtually exhausted, with the NMEs over the last decade having been predominantly "me too" drugs with little, if any, clinically meaningful differences compared with already marketed drugs in the same therapeutic class. Over the last two to three decades, drugs were developed to treat the same set of symptoms treated by earlier drugs, and were based on the same mechanisms of action as their predecessors. Nevertheless, advances were made by "cleaning up" the pharmacology of the older drugs. For example, selective serotonin reuptake inhibitors (SSRIs) were without a doubt "cleaner" versions of their predecessors, the tricyclic antidepressants (TCAs) (Preskorn, 1996a). While their mechanism of antidepressant action was not novel, they did not have the mechanisms responsible for the multiple adverse effects – ranging from nuisance to lethal – of the TCAs. It is fair to say that no psychiatric molecular entities with truly novel mechanisms of action have been marketed for the treatment of schizophrenia, major depression, or anxiety disorders since the early 1960s (Preskorn, 2010). In this regard, the "low hanging fruit" appears to have been thoroughly picked.

Since the newer drugs worked via the same therapeutic mechanism of action as the older drugs, the designs of clinical trials over this period were essentially the same as those used for the original drugs. The advantage of this approach was that it followed a proven pathway to marketing approval by the US Food and Drug Administration. The disadvantage of drug development in recent decades is that the process did not yield novel compounds to address unmet needs in a new way. As most researchers involved with industry and academia believe, this "era" of refining pharmacology is coming to a close, as NMEs targeting specific illnesses are being developed. In fact, CNS drug development may see its first "disease-altering" compounds reach the market over the next 5 to 10 years, with treatments for Alzheimer's dementia currently appearing to be earliest in line for likely approval (Panza *et al.*, 2011).

This shift to developing truly novel compounds is likely to require new trial designs for a variety of reasons. First and foremost, the same "rehashed" study designs that have been used to study older compounds, which had derivative mechanisms of action and acted symptomatically, are not likely to yield meaningful data in the study of truly novel compounds with different mechanisms of action that may be capable of altering the course of the illness. Therefore, it will likely be necessary to revise Phase I studies to achieve a quicker, seamless transition from normal healthy volunteers to participants with the target illness, when the preliminary results warrant such a transition.

Such studies will aim to answer the following questions:

- Is the PK profile of the drug the same in normal healthy volunteers as in the participants with the target illness? There are many examples where the PK profile of a drug differs to a clinically meaningful extent between young healthy and elderly healthy patients.
- Is the dose-response curve in patients with the target illness the same as in young healthy volunteers? For example, a consensus exists that normal healthy volunteers do not tolerate dopamine-2 receptor antagonists (e.g. haloperidol) as well as volunteers with schizophrenia.
- Does the drug cross the blood-brain barrier and does it reach/modulate its desired target to a desired degree?

To address these questions, Phase I studies must be expanded to include data that will allow sponsors to determine whether or not to proceed ("go/no-go" decisions) in a time- and cost-effective fashion.

The same principles apply to early Phase II studies, which are classically concerned with early proof of mechanism (POM), proof of concept (POC), and/or efficacy in the target illness. When developing a study to evaluate efficacy, the measurements used to evaluate specific efficacy endpoints must be carefully examined. If one is examining an NME, scales that were used to evaluate the efficacy of older molecules may not provide meaningful data. For example, the use of the Positive and Negative Syndrome Scale (PANSS) (Kay et al., 1987) to assess efficacy was effective in the late Phase I and early Phase II studies evaluating the pharmacology of "atypical" antipsychotics, which were in essence "re-inventions" of chlorpromazine, which meets all or virtually all of the criteria for "atypicality". Using the PANSS as the primary outcome measure to examine a novel and potentially disease-altering treatment for schizophrenia may not yield meaningful information since the drug may be truly "novel" (Lepping et al., 2011).

Challenges with the traditional approach

Although the traditional process of drug development has led to the successful approval of thousands of currently marketed drugs, it has also resulted in large financial investment in testing compounds that eventually failed to be approved (Paul et al., 2010). As Phase I studies begin to examine truly novel molecules/drugs, many of the "classic" Phase I approaches will no longer be adequate or efficient. Nevertheless, the traditional Phase I single ascending dose (SAD) and multiple ascending dose (MAD) studies have many merits, as was discussed in Part I of this series (Macaluso et al., 2011). The goal in adapting Phase I studies is not to "throw the baby out with the bath water" but instead to keep what works and augment or modify the methodology when it does not address the challenges and demands of central nervous system (CNS) drug development in the twenty-first century.

As discussed, the stages of drug development have traditionally been divided into "learn" and "confirm" phases (Figure 1). Thus, the drug development process leading up to Phase III studies is designed to efficiently identify viable and non-viable compounds, in order to focus resources on the former and discontinue further development of the latter. In contrast, the goal of the "confirm" phase (i.e. Phase III) is to produce substantial evidence that a treatment regimen applied to a particular patient population achieves a specific endpoint that is accepted by regulatory agencies as being efficacious and will yield a sufficient effect size relative to any safety or tolerability concerns to warrant approval (Kraemer *et al.*, 2003). "Confirm" is about hypothesis testing, and the main customers are regulatory agencies (Sheiner, 1997).

Some preliminary questions that Phase I studies may be called on to answer include the following:

- Do the safety, tolerability, and pharmacokinetics (PK) of the drug in normal volunteers generalize to the target population?
- What is the best dose and what is the best dosing schedule to take into Phase II efficacy trials?
- In what subject population (i.e. patients or normal volunteers) and for what indication should the agent be studied?
- What measures should be used to assess the drug's efficacy?

The notion of using Phase I studies solely to explore PK and safety/tolerability in normal volunteers may be both inappropriate and inefficient. Should the earliest exploration of the PK and safety/tolerability of the NME instead be conducted in a population of otherwise healthy individuals with the target psychiatric illness? If that is possible, then one can more meaningfully explore other endpoints, including biomarker surrogates, potentially leading to greater efficiency and cost-effectiveness in the drug development process. Thus, it is important to analyze to what extent data from subjects chosen for early clinical trials can be used to make appropriate inferences about subjects who will eventually be studied in "confirm" trials.

In CNS drug development, sponsors often start with Phase I studies in normal young healthy male volunteers. The reason only male volunteers are used is that the relevant toxicity data necessary to justify testing in women of child-bearing potential may not exist (i.e. that research may not yet have been done) (Spilker, 1991). The main advantages of using normal volunteers are the speed with which subjects can be enrolled and generally lower costs. However, young healthy male subjects may not be good predictors of the PK and/or safety/tolerability of the drug in either females or patients with a particular illness. For instance, the maximum tolerated dose (MTD) of an antipsychotic when tested in normal subjects may be considerably lower than in patients with schizo- phrenia (Gilles and Luthringer, 2007). Hence, the use of otherwise healthy individuals with schizophrenia in Phase I studies might yield more meaningful PK and safety data than studies in normal healthy volunteers, particularly in terms of MTDs. It could therefore be argued that, even in early clinical trials, one should incorporate a seamless transition to participants with the target illness to characterize the dose-response curve in that specific population.

Along these lines, in oncology, individuals diagnosed with cancer are considered a "special population" (Agrawal and Emanuel, 2003). Phase I oncology studies are often conducted in patients rather than normal healthy volunteers for several reasons. First, cancer drugs are often inherently toxic to human cells, so that it may be considered unethical to expose normal healthy volunteers to the potential toxicity of the NME as the first step in its development (Emanuel, 1995). In addition, there is also the potential for an early efficacy signal in individuals who have likely exhausted all available treatments.

In a similar manner, psychiatric patients are also a "special population". As discussed above, doses of drugs that are commonly used in individuals with psychiatric illnesses are often intolerable to normal controls. However, we are also aware of a number of instances in which drugs with a CNS mechanism of action have dose-response curves that are shifted to the left in participants with the target illness compared with the healthy young volunteer population (e.g. dopamine D2 receptor antagonism in patients with Parkinson's disease or muscarinic receptor antagonism in patients with Alzheimer's disease) (Preskorn, personal communication, 2011). These findings mean that the MTD determined in traditional Phase I studies may not be relevant to the dose needed in Phase II efficacy trials. Figure 2 illustrates how dose-response curves can shift either to the right or left in different populations because of pharmacokinetic or pharmacodynamic variables (Preskorn, 1996b).

In addition, the study of CNS drugs in Phase I involves a unique set of challenges that do not apply to other areas of drug investigation, including passage of drugs into the brain; targeting of a specific brain receptor area, transporter, or peptide; and a set of target illnesses that are described syndromically by a set of core symptoms, rather than by a biologically based marker of disease. Finally, certain biomarker endpoints, which are used as a proxy or surrogate for the illness in question, may only be manifested in individuals with the illness (e.g. abnormalities of P50 and P300 evoked potentials in individuals with schizophrenia) (de Visser et al., 2001).

Along the same lines, a potential antipsychotic medication may target certain biological markers such as dopamine D2 or N-methyl-D-aspartate (NMDA) receptors. If that is the case, critical information to establish early on, even in Phase I, would be whether the drug enters the brain and whether it targets a physiologically relevant biomarker endpoint and to what degree (Conn and Roth, 2008). If these conditions are believed to be necessary for the drug to demonstrate efficacy in individuals with the target illness, why not establish such facts as early as possible in the development process? Further, if a drug is intended to target a mechanism that exists only in the diseased population (e.g. a receptor variant), then studying this question early makes good sense in order to determine the ultimate viability of the compound. Thus, the population studied in Phase I may need to be critically assessed (Conn and Roth, 2008). The goal is to "learn" as much as possible in Phase I and II studies to support the best "go/no go" decisions, as well as to inform the design of the "confirm" studies in terms of population, dose(s), and dosing schedule to be studied and endpoints to be measured.

Thus, we propose that the goal of early drug development should be to identify "necessary conditions" which, if not met, would warrant early termination of the drug's development. Even if these conditions are met, the drug may still face future challenges since all "sufficient conditions" must ultimately be met to achieve success. However, the emphasis on identifying "necessary conditions" is helpful in enabling early stopping decisions (Gallo et al., 2006). Establishing safety and tolerability is always necessary, but not generally sufficient if the goal is to develop an effective marketable drug. For example, a drug could be safe and well tolerated in populations of normal volunteers, demonstrating ideal PK, but it may be altogether inadequate as a CNS drug because it does not cross the blood-brain barrier or does not do so sufficiently to establish therapeutic concentrations (i.e. minimal predicted efficacious concentrations) in the brain region of interest. While crossing the blood-brain barrier can be addressed in

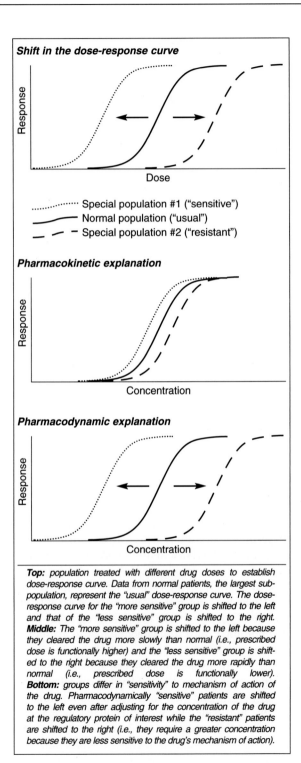

Figure 2. Shifts in dose-response curves in special populations.

preclinical pharmacology, those findings may not predict what happens in humans, nor do they indicate effective target modulation.*

If these types of questions can be addressed early, "go/no-go" decisions can be made safely in a more time- and cost-effective manner, adding a "litmus test" to the usual exploratory endpoints prior to entering the "confirm" phase. If such knowledge can be obtained in Phase I studies, meaningful amounts of time and money can be saved that can potentially be devoted to other compounds or areas of investigation.

A key point is that the approach to early clinical development should be tailored to the needs of the individual program. Studies investigating a first-in-class compound about which little pre-existing knowledge is available will require a different approach than a "me-too" compound whose pharmacokinetic and pharmacodynamic profile is well understood.

Thus, the drug developer must decide on a number of important issues in designing the early studies. For viable compounds, the goal is to establish the correct treatment regimen, patient population, and endpoints to be taken into the "confirm" trials. This information also provides essential feedback on how to optimize follow-up compounds. In light of what has been learned about the NME, can effective target modulation be achieved? Can direct or indirect evidence of efficacy be demonstrated? How can the therapeutic index be optimized relative to the exposure profile (i.e. does a high or low peak/trough ratio exist)?

In terms of dosing, a much more accurate method of determining the MTD is the continuous reassessment method (CRM) (Goodman *et al.*, 1995). The objective of the CRM is to use information gathered in real time to decide on how many more subjects should be allocated to the current dose and to decide what the next dose level should be. In some companies, the CRM has superseded more traditional approaches. The CRM and other adaptive designs will be discussed in greater detail later in this chapter.

In gathering information about dosing, it is valuable to construct a "therapeutic index" (TI), which immediately focuses attention on both efficacy and safety. In early clinical trials, observations about efficacy may be limited to biomarker endpoints, but keeping efficacy in mind will strongly influence the design of these early trials. For instance, if an acceptable safety/tolerability profile cannot be established at exposures that are predicted to be in the minimal efficacious range, then there is no rationale for moving forward. The application of modeling techniques can efficiently establish which treatment regimen can achieve the best TI. Thus, at least three key ingredients must be established as early as possible in the learn phase of the drug development process (Figure 1):

1. Safety and tolerability
2. Pharmacodynamic measures of efficacy (biomarker-based)
3. Pharmacokinetic information relative to items 1 and 2.

To gather information on how to administer the drug, the study should aim to identify the PK profile that will yield the optimal TI.

---

* Most drugs produce their beneficial and adverse effects by altering the functional status of a regulatory protein. Target modulation could, for example, involve a drug acting as an agonist, antagonist, or inverse agonist at a specific receptor. Effective target modulation means having the effect at the target (e.g. agonism or antagonism) necessary to produce the desired clinical effect with minimal adverse effects.

The questions posed above are as provocative as they are practical. If the early stage of the drug development process is not revised so that such questions can be answered efficiently in terms of both time and cost, the future of CNS drug development could be in jeopardy, as excessive dollars will be spent on compounds that are not viable, discouraging companies from developing NMEs and biological agents that may in fact work. In order to better address these questions, we will now explore how adaptive trial designs can streamline this process.

Adaptive trial designs

What makes a trial design adaptive? The main tenet of adaptive trial design is the ability to examine data in "real time" and to "react" or adjust to the new information as the study is ongoing (Gallo *et al.*, 2006). This approach allows a study to be terminated early for futility (i.e. the study is unable to meaningfully test efficacy) or for success earlier than would be possible in traditional nonadaptive trials. The goal is to improve the quality and the speed of decision-making (e.g. the ability to determine which dose and dosing regimen is optimal). Adaptive designs also serve to minimize the number of individuals unnecessarily exposed to compounds that are not viable, because they are either ineffective or unsafe (Krams *et al.*, 2007). On the other hand, there is the potential to stop early for success, ultimately bringing beneficial therapies to patients more quickly. Hence, adaptive trial designs have the potential to produce valid decision-making more quickly, while reducing costs and conserving valuable research resources.

The goal of adaptive designs is to learn from the accumulating trial data and to apply this newly gained knowledge as quickly as possible to optimize the ongoing execution of the study (Krams *et al.*, 2009; Shen *et al.*, 2011). The study design allows for a number of potential modifications, including stopping the trial or increasing the likelihood of patient assignment to the optimal doses in terms of the balance of safety/tolerability and efficacy.

The adaptive approach must start with early study planning and should involve a multidisciplinary group ranging from statisticians to preclinical and clinical scientists as well as clinical operations personnel. This multidisciplinary team must develop an understanding of the specific patient population and appropriate study endpoints. The goal is to integrate real-time learning, including data acquisition, complex randomization schemes, and enhanced drug supply management requirements (Chow and Chang, 2008).

Adaptive designs involve looking at interim data during the course of the trial without having an impact on the trial's validity and integrity. One method of ensuring maintenance of the trial's validity and integrity is to establish the operating characteristics of the design in advance, either analytically or through simulations, and to demonstrate that there is no inflation of type 1 error. Strategic planning teams must plan the setup/function of data monitoring committees and pre-determine the decision tree for making adaptive "changes" to the study design. In addition, a clear process of how early data will be kept confidential must be defined and conceptualized in advance of study operationalization.

Such "real-time" adaptation can involve the following rules (Chow and Chang, 2008):

- Allocation rule (how subjects will be allocated to which treatment arms)
- Sampling rule (how many subjects will be sampled at the next stage)
- Stopping rule (when to stop the trial, for efficacy, safety, and/or futility)
- Decision rule (decisions pertaining to design changes not covered by the previous three rules).

At any stage, the data may be analyzed and next stages redesigned taking into account all available data.

Types of adaptive designs

First-in-human studies – ascending dose escalation designs. Adaptive model-based dose escalation designs, such as the CRM, can be applied to first-in-human and follow-up multiple ascending dose studies (O'Quigley *et al.*, 1990). In contrast to traditional dose escalation designs, adaptive dose escalation designs typically use modeling of the dose-response relationship to help identify the dose range closest to the MTD. These designs may also establish proof of target modulation, typically utilizing biomarker endpoints.

Determining optimal dose. In cases where dose-response is thought to be monotonic, design efficiency can be achieved by starting with the highest tolerated dose and placebo. Pre-determined futility conditions can be included and should force early termination of the study if not met. If futility conditions are not met, the dose-response relationship can be assessed with the goal of determining "optimal dose".

Response adaptive dose-ranging study designs. Dose-response can be evaluated efficiently by using response-adaptive allocation designs in which the trial begins with a greater number of dose levels than are typically included in conventional clinical trials (Gaydos *et al.*, 2006). Instead of using classic pair-wise comparisons, these response adaptive designs include real-time modeling of dose-response data to identify dose levels that fulfill pre-determined set-points. Data are applied immediately and affect the drug dose that future subjects in the study will receive. When futility is met, this may result in discontinuation of non-viable treatment arms or of the entire study.

Now that we have examined the applicability of adaptive trial designs, we will explore the use of biomarkers in clinical trials.

Biomarker endpoints

In an era in which 90% of investigational new drugs fail to make it to market, the use of biomarkers can efficiently and cost-effectively identify NMEs that are unlikely to be viable, with the goal of not wasting any more resources on such NMEs than is necessary to make a valid "no go" decision. If the NME fails to reach its target or to appropriately modulate that target as assessed by a clinically meaningful biomarker, one can make a "no go" decision.

The FDA defines a biomarker as a "measurable characteristic that is an indicator of normal biologic processes, pathogenic processes, and/or response to therapeutic or other interventions" (USDHHS, E15). Commonly used biomarkers in medicine include blood pressure as a predictor of strokes; congestive heart failure and serum cholesterol and triglyceride levels for atherosclerosis; serum glucose for complications of diabetes mellitus; various serum enzyme levels for disease and/or inflammation of various organs (e.g. heart, liver, and pancreas); and QTc interval for the risk of causing torsades de pointes (Chapel *et al.*, 2009). The use of biomarkers in psychiatry has somewhat lagged behind their use in other areas of medicine because of lack of information about the underlying pathophysiology and pathoetiology of psychiatric illnesses. Nevertheless, a number of examples can be cited, including serum prolactin levels as a marker for the degree of dopamine D2 receptor antagonism achieved by a given dose of a given antipsychotic and changes in P50, N100, P300, and mismatched negativity evoked potentials as markers for cognitive impairment associated with schizophrenia (Preskorn *et al.*, 2009).

Most biomarkers are developed via pathway analysis, proteomics, and expression profiles. Researchers must use validated biomarkers that have been compared to already established clinical endpoints (i.e. antipsychotic efficacy). A review of all possible and/or validated biomarkers in psychiatry is beyond the scope of this chapter, and readers are referred to several recently released FDA documents on acceptable biomarkers in clinical trials for a more thorough review (USDHHS, E15, E16, Guidance for industry).

One approach to identifying validated biomarkers that has been the subject of recent attention involves the use of positron emission tomography to examine CNS drug binding to target receptors or interaction with neurotransmitter systems using radio-labeled isotopes (Wong *et al.*, 2009). A now classic example of this approach is dopamine D2 receptor occupancy in the brain. Nevertheless, important limitations exist. Radiolabeled isotopes (e.g. C-11) have a short half-life and must therefore be made on site, which requires a cyclotron and a sophisticated and expensive group of radiochemists. Unless optimal isotopes are used, the brain exposure/concentration may be underestimated when compared to the drug's actual PK (Wong *et al.*, 2009). These technical challenges are being addressed and the application of such imaging to early-phase clinical trials is now one of the tools used in early human testing of an NME. Use of this technology can help determine the doses needed to produce appropriate drug concentration at the desired target in the desired brain regions and appropriate target modulation for optimal therapeutic efficacy.

Only a few indisputable biomarkers exist for any specific psychiatric illness, none of which is currently universally accepted for serious psychiatric illnesses such as schizophrenia, bipolar disorder, and major depression. Nevertheless, considerable work is under way and beginning to bear fruit to establish specific biomarkers that can be helpful in identifying a drug's potential therapeutic efficacy. For example, the use of saccadic eye movements and prolactin response in the development of antipsychotic drugs has been correlated with MTD as well as development of adverse events (de Visser *et al.*, 2001; Sweeney *et al.*, 1997). In fact, more than 80% of all studies utilizing such biomarkers have proven useful in moving the field and NMEs forward (de Visser *et al.*, 2001).

In the area of antidepressant drugs, the Biomarkers for the Rapid Identification of Treatment Effectiveness in Major Depression (BRITE-MD) study showed that pre-frontal lobe activity after 1 week of treatment with escitalopram was correlated with efficacy 7 weeks later (Leuchter *et al.*, 2009). Additional biomarkers in the development of antidepressant drugs include the effect of the drug on rapid eye movement (REM) sleep as well as EEG biomarkers (Steiger and Kimura, 2010). If such a biomarker can be shown to be necessary for drug response in some or all populations, its use early in clinical trial development would be extremely helpful in developing a new antidepressant that also worked via the serotonin pathway.

The biomarkers discussed above were developed for and lend themselves to the development of drugs targeted to treat specific symptoms. While CNS drug development has come a long way, the future is sure to hold new entities that target specific illnesses rather than symptoms. The development of biomarkers for specific illnesses will not only improve the drug development process, but will change psychiatric diagnosis and treatment dramatically from what is accepted orthodoxy today.

Table 1. Key points concerning early-phase drug development studies

Phase I studies
Traditional Phase I studies involve normal volunteers
Single and multiple ascending doses used to determine whether the drug/biologic has appropriate pharmacokinetics and safety/tolerability
Expanded Phase I studies involve volunteers mildly symptomatic with the target illness
Single and multiple ascending doses used to determine whether the drug/biologic has similarly appropriate pharmacokinetics and safety/tolerability and whether the dose-response curves remain the same or shift to the right or left in the target population (Figure 2)
Biomarker may be used to obtain early indication about whether the new drug is likely to be efficacious in individuals more symptomatic with the target illness
Studies in mildly symptomatic volunteers can be done (1) in the same protocol, with a seamless transition from normal volunteers to an approximation of the target population, or (2) in separate protocols
Clinical trial designs
Traditional designs: pre-determined and inflexible protocols that specify what conditions will be studied (e.g. placebo, active comparator, and three fixed doses of the investigational medication) with a pre-determined number of subjects to be enrolled
Adaptive trial designs: design allows for modification of the protocol using pre-specified algorithms and blinded analysis of data in real time. Common modifications that may be made during adaptive trials involve the doses studied, the number of individuals assigned to a given dose, and whether the study is terminated early for either success or failure (Shen *et al.*, 2011)

Conclusion

CNS drug development is rapidly evolving to meet the unique and changing demands of the fields of psychiatry and neurology. To adapt to these unique challenges, Phase I clinical trials must incorporate new principles and methodology to more efficiently identify those drugs that are not viable before they enter late phase (i.e. Phase III) testing. In this way, the traditional approach to Phase I clinical trials is not "wrong" but instead is a starting point that must be modified and amplified to create a "customized" and efficient approach to the development of specific NMEs with truly novel mechanisms of action and the potential to modify disease rather than simply providing symptomatic relief. Key points covered in this chapter are summarized in Table 1. We have proposed that the potential target population be examined in Phase I trials after studies with normal volunteers have been completed in order to increase the efficiency and precision of decisions made based on Phase I data. The use of an adaptive design to examine data and modify the study in real time may also promote time- and cost-efficient identification of NMEs that have the characteristics necessary to be successful in "confirm" stages of drug development research. Finally, we discussed how use of biomarkers as surrogate endpoints can be incorporated into early clinical trials to determine if a drug modulates the appropriate targets, which, in turn, enhances the likelihood of demonstrating efficacy in the "confirm" phase of clinical testing.

References

Agrawal, M. and Emanuel, E. J. (2003). Ethics of Phase I oncology studies: Reexamining the arguments and data. *J Am Med Assoc*, 290, 1075–82.

Arbuck, S. G. (1996). Workshop on Phase I study design. Ninth NCI/EORTC New Drug Development Symposium, Amsterdam, March 12, *Ann Oncol*, 7, 567–73.

Chapel, S., Hutmacher, M. M., Haig, G., *et al.* (2009). Exposure-response analysis in patients with schizophrenia to assess the effect of asenapine on QTc prolongation. *J Clin Pharmacol*, 49, 1297–308.

Chow, S. C. and Chang, M. (2008). Adaptive design methods in clinical trials – A review. *Orphanet J Rare Dis*, 3, 11.

Conn, P. J. and Roth, B. L. (2008). Opportunities and challenges of psychiatric drug discovery: Roles for scientists in academic, industry, and government settings. *Neuropsychopharmacology*, 33, 2048–60.

Crane, M. and Newman, M. C. (2000). What level of effect is a no observed effect? *Environ Toxicol Chem*, 19, 516–19.

Dragalin, V. (2006). Terminology and classification of adaptive designs. *Drug Info J*, 40, 425–35.

Emanuel, E. J. (1995). A Phase I trial on the ethics of Phase I trials. *J Clin Oncol*, 13, 1049–51.

Gallo, P., Chuang-Stein, C., Dragalin, V., *et al.* (2006). Executive summary of the PhRMA Working Group on adaptive designs in clinical drug development. *J Biopharmaceutical Statistics*, 16, 275–83.

Gaydos, B., Krams, M., Perevozskaya, I., *et al.* (2006). Adaptive dose-response studies. *Drug Info J*, 40, 451–61.

Gilles, C. and Luthringer, R. (2007). Pharmacological models in healthy volunteers: Their use in the clinical development of psychotropic drugs. *J Psychopharmacol*, 21, 272–82.

Goodman, S. N., Zahurak, M. L., and Piantadosi, S. (1995). Some practical improvements in the continual reassessment method for Phase I studies. *Stat Med*, 14, 1149–61.

Kaitin, K. I. (2010). Deconstructing the drug development process: The new face of innovation. *Clin Pharmacol Ther*, 87, 356–61.

Kay, S. R., Fiszbein, A., and Opler, L. A. (1987). The Positive and Negative Syndrome Scale (PANSS) for schizophrenia. *Schizophrenia Bull*, 13, 261–76.

Kraemer, H. C., Morgan, G. A., Leech, N. L., *et al.* (2003). Measures of clinical significance. *J Am Acad Child Adolesc Psych*, 42, 1524–9.

Krams, M., Burman, C. F., Dragalin, V., *et al.* (2007). Adaptive designs in clinical drug development: Opportunities, challenges, and scope reflections following PhRMA's November 2006 workshop. *J Biopharm Stat*, 17, 957–64.

Krams, M., Sharma, S., Dragalin, V., *et al.* (2009). Adaptive approaches in clinical drug development: Opportunities and challenges in design and implementation. *Pharmaceut Med*, 23, 139–48.

Lepping, P., Sambhi, R. S., Whittington, R., *et al.* (2011). Clinical relevance of findings in trials of antipsychotics: Systematic review. *Brit J Psychiat*, 198, 341–5.

Leuchter, A. F., Cook, I. A., Marangell, L. B., *et al.* (2009). Comparative effectiveness of biomarkers and clinical indicators for predicting outcomes of SSRI treatment in major depressive disorder: Results of the BRITE-MD study. *Psychiat Res*, 169, 124–31.

Macaluso, M., Krams, M., and Preskorn, S. H. (2011). Phase I trials: From traditional to newer approaches. Part I. *J Psychiatr Pract*, 17, 200–3.

McConnell, E. E. (1989). The maximum tolerated dose: the debate. *J Am Coll Toxicol*, 8, 1115–20.

Meinert, C. L. and Tonascia, S. (1986). *Clinical Trials: Design, Conduct, and Analysis* (p. 3). New York: Oxford University Press.

O'Quigley, J., Pepe, M., and Fisher, L. (1990). Continual reassessment method: A practical design for Phase I clinical trials in cancer. *Biometrics*, 46, 33–48.

Panza, F., Frisardi, V., Imbimbo, B. P., *et al.* (2011). Monoclonal antibodies against b-amyloid (Ab) for the treatment of Alzheimer's disease: the Ab target at a crossroads. *Expert Opin Biol Ther*, 11, 679–86.

Paul, S. M., Mytelka, D. S., Dunwiddie, C. T., *et al.* (2010). How to improve R&D productivity: The pharmaceutical industry's grand challenge. *Nat Rev Drug Discov*, 9, 203–14.

Preskorn, S. H. (1996a). How SSRIs as a group differ from TCAs. In: Preskorn, S. (Ed.), *Clinical Pharmacology of SSRI's*. Wichita, KS: Professional Communications, Inc.. http://www.preskorn.com/books/ssri_open.html. Accessed January 10, 2011.

Preskorn, S. H. (1996b). If lack of concentration didn't cause the fall, what did? *J Pract Psychiat Behav Health*, 2, 364–7.

Preskorn, S. H. (2010). CNS drug development: Part I: The early period of CNS drugs. *J Psychiatr Pract*, 16, 334–39.

Preskorn, S., D'Empaire, I., Baker, B., *et al.* (2009). EVP-6124, an alpha-7 nicotinic agonist produces normalizing effects on evoked response biomarkers and cognition in patients with chronic schizophrenia on stable antipsychotic therapy. Poster presented at the 2009 American College of Neuropsychopharmacology meeting, Hollywood, FL, December.

Sheiner, L. B. (1997). Learning versus confirming in clinical drug development. *Clin Pharmacol Ther*, 61, 275–91.

Shen, J., Preskorn, S., Dragalin, V., *et al.* (2011). How adaptive trial designs can increase efficiency in psychiatric drug development: A case study. *Innov Clin Neurosci*, 8, 26–34.

Spilker, B. (1991). *Guide to Clinical Trials*. Baltimore: Lippincott Williams & Wilkins.

Steiger, A. and Kimura, M. (2010). Wake and sleep EEG provide biomarkers in depression. *J Psychiatr Res*, 44, 242–52.

Sweeney, J. A., Bauer, K. S., Keshavan, M. S., *et al.* (1997). Adverse effects of risperidone on eye movement activity: A comparison of risperidone and haloperidol in antipsychotic-naive schizophrenic patients. *Neuropsychopharmacology*, 16, 217–28.

US Department of Health and Human Services, Food and Drug Administration (FDA), Center for Drug Evaluation and Research (CDER), Center for Biologics Evaluation and Research (CBER). E15 definitions for genomic biomarkers, pharmacogenetics, genomic data, and sample coding categories, April 2008 (available at www.fda.gov/downloads/RegulatoryInformation/Guidances/ucm129296.pdf, accessed July 7, 2011).

US Department of Health and Human Services, FDA, CDER, CBER. E16 genomic biomarkers related to drug response: Context, structure, and format of qualification submissions (draft guidance) (available at www.fda.gov/downloads/Drugs/GuidanceComplianceRegulatoryInformation/Guidances/UCM174433.pdf, accessed July 7, 2011).

US Department of Health and Human Services, FDA, CDER, CBER. Guidance for industry: Pharmacogenomic data submissions (available at www.fda.gov/downloads/Drugs/GuidanceComplianceRegulatoryInformation/Guidances/ucm079849.pdf, accessed July 7, 2011).

de Visser, S. J., van der Post, J., Pieters, M. S., *et al.* (2001). Biomarkers for the effects of antipsychotic drugs in healthy volunteers. *Br J Clin Pharmacol*, 512, 119–32.

Wong, D. F., Tauscher, J., and Gründer, G. (2009). The role of imaging in proof of concept for CNS drug discovery and development. *Neuropsychopharmacology*, 34, 187–203.

Phase II development and the path to personalized medicine in CNS disease

Douglas E. Feltner and Kenneth R. Evans

Introduction and general issues

Phase II is a critical period during drug development. Failure of novel drug candidates occurs commonly, with lack of efficacy being the usual reason. In this chapter, we will provide information to assist drug developers in progressing through Phase II with the highest likelihood of success, or alternatively, to reach a stop development decision, where that is necessary, as cheaply as possible. We first address general Phase II clinical development issues and pitfalls and the relationship of Phase II to the preceding and subsequent phases of development, and then focus on the new issues introduced into Phase II development by the emergence of personalized medicine.

During Phase II, the first evidence of efficacy is generally obtained in subjects with the disease of interest, the clinical therapeutic index is roughed out, the doses to study in Phase III are defined, and the safety database is expanded to support Phase III. More broadly, further safety toxicology, formulation, and commercial work are done to prepare for Phase III.

While team enthusiasm is often focused on whether the drug candidate will have efficacy in the indication, much is still unknown about the safety of the drug candidate in Phase II. Medical safety monitoring must be vigilant to quickly detect any safety problem so that study subjects are protected and are appropriately informed as soon as possible of any risks of participating in the study.

Success in Phase II is supported by all of the prior preclinical and clinical work. Preparation for Phase II begins with the appropriate matching of drug target, method of drug modulation of target, and patient population; the preparation continues with identification of a small molecule with appropriate chemical and pharmaceutical properties, development and execution of an adequate plan to obtain a proof-of-mechanism, adequate preclinical safety toxicology to support dosing in Phase II, and finally initial demonstration of safety, tolerability, and human pharmacokinetics in Phase I. All of this activity provides information about the properties of the drug candidate for Phase II, including both the potential benefits and the potential problems that will need to be further evaluated.

The initial demonstration of safety and tolerability in Phase I may be completed in healthy volunteers or subjects with the disorder of interest. Phase I is usually completed in adult healthy volunteers for most disorders. Studies of potential drugs for schizophrenia and Alzheimer's disease often study subjects with the disorder in the multiple rising dose tolerance study, because these subjects may be more or less tolerant of unintended drug effects, depending also on mechanism (Cutler and Sramek, 2000; Cutler, 2001). During Phase I, the

Essential CNS Drug Development, ed. A. Kalali, Sheldon Preskorn, J. Kwentus, and Stephen M. Stahl. Published by Cambridge University Press. © Cambridge University Press 2012.

maximum tolerated single and multiple doses should be defined, so that potential safety and tolerability problems can be better anticipated later in development, where the larger number of exposures in more biologically diverse subjects will result in a wider diversity of responses to the drug candidate. Further, identification of the maximum tolerated multiple dose is a necessary part of understanding whether the mechanistic hypothesis can be tested. Standard pharmacokinetic parameters will also be determined and $t_{1/2}$ used to assist in defining dose frequency.

Bioequivalence (BE), food effect (FE), and drug-drug interaction (DDI) studies may or may not be required prior to Phase II. The timing of these studies will depend on the consequences of the result obtained, the likelihood that a problem may exist, and the philosophy of the drug developer. For example, if the risk of a DDI is low, or a moderate DDI is considered acceptable for that mechanism and indication, then the study can be delayed until after the first efficacy study. On the other hand, if a large DDI is likely, and is unacceptable for that mechanism or indication, or would require additional safety monitoring in Phase II, then the study should be conducted prior to initiating the first Phase II efficacy study. The drug developer should remember when advancing molecules into development that have a reasonable chance of carrying significant or unacceptable DDI, FE, or safety risks, that these drug candidates will require higher costs and often lengthier development tracks to assess these risks, and this should be weighed against bringing forward alternative candidates in the portfolio (if alternatives exist).

It is critical that the drug developer define the central nervous system (CNS) exposure, receptor occupancy, and pharmacodynamic (biomarker) effect required to be certain that the mechanistic hypothesis, rather than just the molecule, is tested. These parameters should be derived from the evidence that most strongly suggests efficacy, whether data from several animal models for a molecule with an unprecedented mechanism of action, or data from a clinically available drug, if the mechanism is precedented. For an unprecedented mechanism, the preclinical data should be related to one another and to animal models of efficacy with a pharmacokinetic-pharmacodynamic (PKPD) model to better quantify the desired effects to be achieved in the clinic. Prior to Phase II, adequate central nervous system exposure and/or receptor occupancy as well as appropriate pharmacodynamic activity should then be demonstrated at a safe and well-tolerated multiple dose in the clinic to verify that the mechanistic hypothesis will be tested in Phase II (Figure 1). Obtaining proof-of-mechanism prior to Phase II allows the sponsoring organization: (1) to save resources by stopping prior to the Phase II efficacy study, if the molecule is not able to test the mechanistic hypothesis; (2) to confidently stop pursuing the mechanistic hypothesis with backup molecules for the studied indication if a negative result is obtained in Phase II; and (3) to qualify the molecule as able to test the mechanistic hypothesis for other CNS indications.

General approaches to Phase IIa and Phase II decision-making

Design of the first efficacy study (sometimes obfuscatingly referred to as a Proof-of-Concept (POC) study) will depend on many factors, including cost, time, whether the mechanism is known to be effective in the chosen indication, and other organizational issues. One can view the first efficacy study as buying a limited amount of information to establish with a desired degree of precision that the drug candidate will have the efficacy and safety properties of a successful drug. Hence, the amount and type of information that

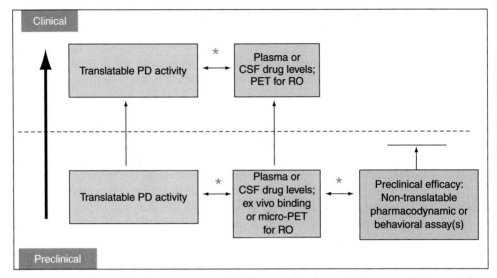

Figure 1. General example for demonstrating translatable proof-of-mechanism. In this generalized example for proving that one is testing the mechanistic hypothesis in the clinic, the strongest preclinical evidence of efficacy, which in this case is not directly demonstrable in humans, is related to receptor occupancy (RO), drug exposure, and a translatable pharmacodynamic (PD) measure using exposure-response models (*). Quantitative criteria for the translatable PD activity, drug exposure, and receptor occupancy are set based on these relationships to the preclinical efficacy signal. Translatable PD activity, drug exposure, and RO are then measured in the clinic to determine whether the mechanism can be tested in a human efficacy study.

one obtains in the first efficacy study should be sufficient to make a clear decision on whether to invest in larger Phase IIb or, in a few limited cases, Phase III studies.

A key factor in determining the design of the first efficacy study will be the confidence in likelihood of the drug actually being efficacious. For drugs with unprecedented mechanisms of action, confidence will often be low, and methods to allow the minimal spend to reach the next decision point should generally be employed.

Information that increases confidence in likelihood of finding clinical efficacy and an adequate therapeutic index (TI) for an unprecedented mechanism are: a wide TI in toxicology studies; concordance of data from several different animal models and other sources pointing toward a similar efficacious concentration/required receptor occupancy; human data supporting the mechanistic hypothesis (e.g. the target is involved in the molecular pathophysiology of the disorder) or genetic (genome-wide association study) data indicating that the target confers risk for the disorder. A strong demonstration of proof-of-mechanism in Phase I with a large TI is especially helpful. The preclinical data for some indications, animal polysomnography data for a proposed insomnia drug or minimal electroshock data for a proposed anti-epileptic, for example, will be more predictive of efficacy in the clinic than data for other indications, such as data from animal models of cognition for a drug proposed to treat cognitive deficits in schizophrenia.

The desired effect size on the primary efficacy measure should be identified a priori and alternative study designs should be examined to determine how efficiently they can provide information necessary for decision-making. Quantitative decision criteria, with the probability of making a correct/incorrect decision based on assumptions of different true drug effect sizes, should be determined, and an agreement reached on the acceptable decision

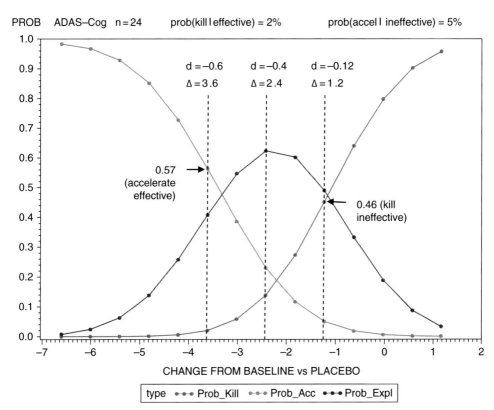

Figure 2. In this example of a first, small efficacy study in Alzheimer's disease, the desired drug-placebo difference (effective drug) on the ADAS-cog outcome measure is 3.6 points (effect size −0.6). A drug-placebo difference of 1.2 (or less) is clearly unacceptable (ineffective). The acceptable probability of advancing an ineffective drug is set at 5%, and the acceptable probability of stopping an effective drug is set at 2%. Given the variability of the ADAS-cog (standard deviation = 6), if the true effect of the drug candidate is 3.6 points, with a sample size of 24 in a 2 x 2 crossover design, there is a 57% probability of advancing an effective drug candidate, a 41% chance of ending up uncertain, and a 2% chance of stopping an effective drug candidate. The probability of stopping an ineffective drug candidate (true drug-placebo difference 1.2 points) is 46%, the probability of ending up uncertain is 49%, and the probability of advancing an ineffective drug candidate is 5%. One can create and examine similar graphical displays for various sample sizes, setting various acceptable probabilities for advancing an ineffective drug or stopping an effective drug, to facilitate getting agreement on the decision rules for the study and to determine the size of investment to make. Probabilities for correct and incorrect decision-making for true drug effects between 1.2 and 3.6 points can also be determined (e.g. 2.4 points is shown). See plate section for color version.

criteria (Figure 2). Determining quantitative criteria for stopping versus continuing drug development after the first efficacy study is critical to mitigating the various forms of bias that influence decision-making in drug development. In developing these decision criteria, it is important to use all of the available information. Including this information in a quantitative model, termed "Model-based Drug Development", can be very helpful in focusing teams on key questions and building consensus on decision criteria (Lalonde *et al.*, 2007; Ouellet *et al.*, 2009).

Study design features: randomization, blinding, active and placebo controls

In the past, small open-label studies have been recommended as a method to get initial efficacy and safety information. Because of the potential for bias in the assessment and interpretation of drug effects in CNS clinical trials, randomization, blinding, and placebo controls should always be used when assessing the efficacy of a CNS drug candidate.

Unfortunately, for reasons that are widely speculated upon but not well understood, drugs known to be active do not always demonstrate efficacy signals different from placebo in CNS clinical trials (Feltner et al., 2009). Therefore, it is generally necessary to include an active control in Phase II studies to demonstrate assay sensitivity. A lack of assay sensitivity has been a particular concern in antidepressant and anxiolytic trials, where effect sizes of approved drugs have been small to moderate and variable. However, a concern about improvement on placebo and its impact on assay sensitivity certainly extends to all trials that use subjective outcome measures, and also may extend to more seemingly objective measures (Kemeny et al., 2007). Active controls can also be useful for obtaining a preliminary estimate of relative effect sizes in indications such as insomnia (utilizing polysomnography), where a greater precision in the estimate of effect size can be obtained with relatively fewer subjects. Inclusion of an active control, however, will increase time and cost to reach the next decision point, and is thus sometimes a point of contentious discussion.

While open-label data should not be used to argue that a drug candidate has efficacy, an additional open-label or controlled study is sometimes needed during Phase I or II to answer a safety question. In some cases, this will need to be done in the patient population, though many questions can be answered in healthy volunteers prior to Phase II. For example, a question regarding QTc prolongation or hepato-toxicity may arise in the single or multiple dose tolerance studies, and more subjects may need to be exposed to better define whether the problem really exists, the severity of the problem, and the exposures that are both safe and otherwise acceptable. Safe exposures can then be compared to the projected efficacious exposures obtained from human mechanistic (biomarker, receptor occupancy) data to determine whether a therapeutic index is likely to exist and to make a decision to continue or to stop development.

It is important to emphasize that if a specific safety issue has arisen that needs clarification, it should be addressed quickly with a well-designed study. Depending on the cost and time required, the safety question might be addressed within a primary efficacy study, but one should not compromise getting a clear answer to a primary safety question that if present could stop development by misfitting it into a study optimized to ask an efficacy question.

Operational considerations: number and selection of clinical study sites

Given that the first efficacy study will have a relatively small number of subjects, preferably, a relatively small number (e.g. 4–12) of sites should be used. This number allows for selection of the best sites and closer and more effective site monitoring, while still providing confidence in the results provided by multicenter data. Unfortunately, blinded, randomized, single-center studies of CNS drugs do not always replicate in multicenter follow-up studies, perhaps because the blinding was ineffective and the investigator's unintended positive bias is allowed to operate on the results, so that multicenter data are needed to provide adequate confidence to proceed. Indeed, it may still be possible in using this small number of sites yet multicenter approach to get a false positive Phase IIa result, as probably occurred for an NK1 antagonist tested as an antidepressant (Keller et al., 2006), though this is uncommon.

Both quantitative and qualitative measures can be used to evaluate clinical study sites. Quantitative measures, including on-time delivery of promised activities (IRB approvals, subject recruitment), subject retention in study, number of protocol deviations, instances where GCPs were not clearly followed, and others are helpful in avoiding the worst sites. Adequate training, and experience of study personnel with the disorder and outcome measures being used, are essential. The conscientiousness of site personnel and lack of bias in applying study criteria to patient selection and primary ratings are critical for conducting a successful study. Despite their importance, these qualitative variables are less commonly assessed, perhaps because they are more difficult to measure.

Study sponsors should be aware that the site personnel who will conduct the study do change over time, and past results may not be predictive of future performance, even for well-established sites.

Dose selection

In addition to maximum tolerated dose data from Phase I, mechanistic pharmacodynamic/biomarker data, receptor occupancy data, and projections of efficacious drug concentrations are extremely useful for defining the dose or doses to be studied in the first efficacy study. Pharmacodynamic (PD) activity that is known from animal data or from a marketed precedented drug to co-occur with doses that are efficacious in the model can be used to identify a likely efficacious clinical dose of the drug candidate. Human in vivo receptor occupancy, determined by PET, can identify the occupancy associated with the translated PD activity, and greater confidence can be obtained in dose selection when the translated PD activity occurs at similar receptor occupancies in animal and man. Human in vivo receptor occupancy measurements can be especially helpful for G-protein-coupled antagonists, where occupancy in the range of 60–90% will likely be required for efficacy (Grimwood and Hartig, 2009).

Whether one or more than one (typically two) dose should be studied in the first efficacy study must be addressed. This choice will be influenced by the certainty of the prediction of the efficacious dose, the need for more or less extensive information on therapeutic index at this early stage of development, confidence in the likelihood of efficacy, concerns about an inverted U-shaped dose-response curve, and other more practical considerations.

Where insufficient understanding of mechanistic activity and estimated efficacious drug concentration has been generated prior to the first efficacy study, a broad range of doses may be tolerated and may need to be considered for assessment of efficacy. In this unfavorable circumstance, one could choose to simply study the maximum tolerated dose. Alternatively, if the indication has appropriate characteristics, an adaptive trial that initially studies many doses and plans to stop randomization to those that are ineffective can be employed (Krams *et al.*, 2003). One should not, however, conduct studies with a large number of dose groups in indications where placebo response is a significant concern, because these designs can increase expectancy of benefit, increase placebo response, decrease assay sensitivity, and result in uninformative trials (Sinyor *et al.*, 2010).

Depending on the indication, the shape of the dose-response curve may not be known with any precision prior to the exposure of large numbers of subjects in Phase III. This is true for depression, anxiety, schizophrenia, and bipolar disorder. Insomnia is an exception, where PSG can be used in a small number of subjects to define rather precisely the dose-response curve for efficacy and tolerability endpoints, and a clinical utility for each dose of the drug candidate can be determined (Ouellet *et al.*, 2009).

As mentioned above, an inverted U-shaped dose-response curve may be raised as a possibility. Typically, this is raised as a concern by discovery scientists and unfortunately just as often dismissed without consideration by experienced drug developers with the view that inverted U-shaped dose-response curves do not exist and even if they do, they are not drugs. Though inverted U-shaped dose-response curves are probably rare in the clinic, these concerns should instead be met with an evaluation of the strength of the data supporting the inverted U, preferably well before the drug candidate reaches the clinic. In addition, the breadth of the peak of the proposed inverted U relative to the PK variability of the drug candidate must be evaluated to determine whether it will be possible to find a dose that will place the majority of subjects at near-peak efficacy. If the range of doses proposed to provide maximal efficacy is quite small and the PK variability of the candidate is relatively large, it may not be possible for most subjects to receive a near maximally efficacious dose, unless dosing is directed by sampling plasma drug concentrations.

Dose frequency

Dosing frequency is usually determined from the plasma pharmacokinetic half-life ($t_{1/2}$) with the dosing interval approximately equal to the $t_{1/2}$. Thus, a drug candidate with a 12 hour half-life would be tested with twice-daily dosing in the first efficacy study. The duration of central pharmacodynamic effects can also provide useful information for determining dosing frequency. Dosing close to the $t_{1/2}$ helps to minimize peak-to-trough variation in drug concentration, while maintaining free plasma concentrations above the projected efficacious concentrations. Minimizing variation in peak to trough concentrations may be helpful in reducing some adverse events, because at least some tolerability problems are related to peak plasma concentrations. The rate at which drug concentration increases to a maximum is also important for tolerability, with the effects associated with faster increases in drug concentration being perceived as stronger effects. Commercial concerns sometimes compel less frequent dosing than is supported by the $t_{1/2}$, and this may lead to testing a larger, less well-tolerated dose to maintain a minimal plasma concentration with less frequent dosing. When clinical efficacy is unknown for the mechanism, additional dosing regimens should not be added into the first efficacy study. The optimal dose frequency should be tested. Alternative dosing frequencies can be tested in Phase IIb, or if pharmacokinetic data and modeling suggest this is unlikely to be successful, controlled-release formulation work can be initiated.

While free brain drug concentrations are of primary interest, free plasma drug concentrations can be a useful surrogate for free brain concentrations so long as the drug candidate has been shown to be in free equilibrium between the brain and plasma compartments (preferably in a nonhuman primate, rather than rodent species) and is not a substrate for the P-glycoprotein transporter.

While the approach of maintaining a minimal drug concentration above the projected efficacious concentration throughout the dosing period is generally taken, the hypothesis that continuous receptor occupancy may not be necessary, and in fact may be detrimental, is sometimes raised. With agonist drug candidates, the concern is that continuous receptor occupancy may produce tolerance to the intended effect. Some drug candidates can produce various forms of receptor desensitization that might also be hypothesized to mitigate clinical efficacy. If the development of tolerance to intended drug effect is thought to be a concern due to compelling data, then a treatment group with a dosing schedule with less frequent dosing to allow for recovery of receptor sensitivity can be included or even substituted for the standard approach. The dosing frequency to test should be derived from preclinical data and from human biomarker evidence of the development of and recovery from tolerance to intended effect. To be compelling, there should be a correspondence of data demonstrating the phenomenon of tolerance from several sources, as well as mechanistic data providing an explanatory basis for why the tolerance is occurring (e.g. receptor desensitization due to internalization, receptor phosphorylation). Phenomena such as development of tolerance create a substantial challenge to the drug candidate and the risk of failure is likely high, as one must presumably dose frequently enough to provide efficacy, but not so frequently as to produce tolerance, and the ability to predict what the appropriate frequency would be and the translatability of information from preclinical models and human biomarker data is highly uncertain.

Selection of indication

Matching the right target for the right indication is undoubtedly the most difficult challenge facing CNS drug discoverers and developers. The initial indication for a particular drug candidate is usually chosen very early during the discovery process, often before lead development. The target will be paired with one or more indications when the discovery project is initiated, and generally pared down to a single indication as data are developed and the project advances. While the choice of indication may be influenced by both scientific and commercial factors, the indication chosen should be the one that gives the drug the best chance to demonstrate efficacy with acceptable initial safety (acceptable varies by indication), allowing for an initial demonstration of value for the drug candidate. This decision should have input from specialist clinicians familiar with the indications under consideration.

Inclusion of exploratory measures in the first efficacy study can be useful in identifying additional indications where the drug candidate may be of benefit. Data from the Profile of Mood States from a gabapentin epilepsy study, for example, were used as an important part of the support for testing gabapentin and later pregabalin in the anxiety disorder indications (Dimond et al., 1996).

Indication selection, matching targets to patients, can be facilitated by collecting appropriate genetic or other biological information about the proposed subject population, and assuring that the biology of the subjects is matched to the drug candidate's proposed mechanism. Approaches to personalized medicine and their impact on Phase II are discussed in detail later in this chapter.

Phase IIb

If decision criteria to advance the drug candidate are met following the first efficacy study, a larger Phase IIb efficacy and safety study is usually initiated. Additional first efficacy studies in additional indications may also be conducted. The primary scientific goals of Phase IIb are to refine estimates of TI and dose, and to expand the safety database in preparation for Phase III. Further, the Phase IIb study confirms and further defines the initial efficacy signal. A more comprehensive commercial valuation is done and medical, pharmaceutical, toxicological, and regulatory plans for Phase III and commercial marketing of the drug candidate are constructed in greater detail. This planning is an iterative process and is re-evaluated as each study completes and new information about the safety, efficacy, and other properties of the drug candidate emerge.

A number of additional clinical studies are conducted in Phase IIb if needed. DDI, food effect, bioequivalence, thorough QT, and abuse potential studies may be done during Phase IIb, if they clarify issues that could significantly impact Phase III study designs, the Phase III development plan, commercial value, or product label.

The increased amount of efficacy information across a wider range of doses helps to refine the dose-response curve, and to identify the dose or doses to carry forward into Phase III. The precision with which the dose-response curve can be characterized by the end of Phase IIb will depend on the number of exposures, the effect size, the PK variability of the drug candidate, and the range of doses studied. The precision for indications with small to medium and variable effect sizes, such as depression and anxiety disorders, will often be poor, requiring that a range of doses be studied in Phase III. Collecting a sufficient number of PK samples to expand understanding of the exposure-response relationships can be helpful in increasing the precision of choice of doses to use in Phase III. Exposure-response information on safety measures (Chapel *et al.*, 2009) can often improve the precision of the estimated therapeutic index and better clarify thresholds for stopping/continuing drug development.

The number of subjects exposed to multiple doses of the drug candidate increases significantly during Phase IIb. The increase in exposures helps to identify any uncommon major safety problems prior to a significant Phase III investment, providing sufficient confidence to enter Phase III. There is no set rule on the number of exposures needed to enter Phase III, but, in addition to the healthy volunteer exposures, usually several hundred subjects with the disorder will have been exposed to multiple doses.

Accelerating Phase II development: combining or skipping phases

Two methods for speeding up development involve variations on approaches to Phase II. In unusual circumstances, it may be possible to conduct only one Phase II efficacy study before progressing to Phase III. If one has a substantial amount of data for an approved drug with an identical mechanism of action, this information can be used along with a single, larger than usual Phase IIa study to provide sufficient information to progress to Phase III. PET data on target occupancy for the marketed drug and the drug candidate or comparative PD (biomarker) data can be especially useful for dose selection in this circumstance. One has to be confident that the mechanisms of the new drug candidate and marketed drug are really identical, including any relevant secondary pharmacology. With sufficient PKPD modeling and sufficient exposures in Phase II, this approach can be successful, though may require studying more doses in Phase III, if the dose projections lack precision.

A second approach to accelerating drug development involves proposing to do a "combined Phase IIb/3" clinical study. In essence, this approach promises to do Phase IIb dose ranging, conduct an interim analysis, use the interim analysis for the End-of-Phase II meeting with the FDA and to trigger Phase III investments, possibly adapt the trial by reducing the number of dose arms after the interim, and finally complete the study and have the highly powered dose group satisfy requirements for regulators to declare it sufficient as a demonstration of one of the two required efficacy studies. In practice, it is not practical to shield the clinical study team and other individuals at the sponsor from the FDA discussions which involve the interim results, so that if one wants to trigger FDA discussions and then Phase III investments from a Phase IIb study interim analysis, the study is unlikely to be anything more than supportive of efficacy.

Biomarkers and personalized medicine

Patients who meet the diagnostic criteria for almost any given disease will show a high degree of heterogeneity in treatment outcome, disease onset and aggressiveness, and/or in the specific combinations of symptoms that are manifested. This heterogeneity can pose significant challenges to the development of new drugs since historically there has been no way to define which patients require alternative therapeutic approaches. The result has been overly inclusive study populations, poor signal-to-noise ratios and development failure even for drugs that were effective in a subset of patients. Indeed, even drugs with sufficiently robust efficacy profiles to achieve regulatory approval are not effective in all patients, and heterogeneity of response remains a critical issue in the clinic. Faced with a non-responsive patient, clinicians have little choice but to experiment with several different medications in order to identify the most effective approach, thereby exposing the patient to unnecessary side effects while delaying the initiation of effective treatment. This increases the costs to society not just in terms of wasted medications and medical resources, but because delaying the onset of effective therapy can negatively impact the long-term outcomes for the patient (Killackey and Yung, 2007).

Fortunately, advances in medicine, particularly in the fields of genomics, proteomics, and other "omic" methodologies, are changing this paradigm. These technologies have dramatically increased our understanding of the biological underpinnings of disease heterogeneity, giving drug developers new avenues with which to identify those patients who are predisposed to respond to a given therapeutic approach. Such "personalized medicines" should be more likely to succeed during development, while improving outcomes when the drugs reach the clinic. Moreover, these advances are changing our understanding of disease at a fundamental level.

Advances in the treatment of breast cancer are an important illustration of the personalized medicine paradigm. The Her2Neu (Human Epidermal Growth Factor) protein is overexpressed in about 25% of breast cancer patients, a subset that has historically been associated with poor outcomes. Trastuzumab, a monoclonal antibody, was developed to target this protein and has been subsequently proven efficacious in about 45% of those patients testing positive for Her2Neu overexpression (Slamon *et al.*, 2001). Consequently, Her2Neu testing is now routinely used to determine treatment options in breast cancer. Trastuzumab is therefore an interesting example of the power of personalized medicine approaches, but also shows that even with highly targeted therapies there will be heterogeneity in response.

Biomarker-based therapies such as trastuzumab in breast cancer or imatinib in chronic myeloid leukemia are in many respects special cases, since the biomarkers used to predict responsiveness are also the therapeutic targets and were obviously well known prior to the onset of clinical trials. For most drugs available in the clinic, however, markers of response will not be identified until retrospective biomarker discovery studies can be conducted on samples drawn from completed efficacy studies. In some cases the task will be easier since the targets for such research may be obvious. Response to serotonin reuptake inhibitors (SSRIs) in Major Depressive Disorder (MDD), for example, has been linked to polymorphisms of the monoamine transporter gene, which in turn appear to be dependent on other variables such as ethnic background and gender (Huezo-Diaz *et al.*, 2009; Kim *et al.*, 2006). Further, for many drugs the assessment of markers related to the mechanism of action will not by itself explain the variability in response. For example, mutations within cytochrome P450 genes (which produce enzymes responsible for the metabolism of many drugs) can severely impact response rates and adverse events effects profiles. Indeed, 62% of FDA-approved drug labels that incorporate pharmacogenomics language pertain to cytochrome P450 polymorphisms (Frueh *et al.*, 2008). Similarly, alterations in biological systems lying up- or downstream from the mechanism of action of a drug might significantly impact the utility of a given therapy, but unless preclinical models can comprehensively mimic the complexity of human biology, such research can only be conducted in association with clinical trials. In other words, the early personalized medicine success stories, while exciting, are nevertheless relatively simple examples in a complex and challenging new field.

Ideally, response-associated markers will be identified prior to the onset of pivotal clinical trials such that enriched populations are incorporated into Phase III and, ultimately, into clinical practice. However, the integration of biomarker research into Phase II creates numerous challenges in terms of study design, cost, analysis techniques, and timelines. Nevertheless, elements of biomarker research have become routine for many pharmaceutical companies and as technologies, methods, and reliability improve, these research activities will only increase. It is all the more important therefore that drug developers fully understand both the shortcomings and power of these "bleeding edge" technologies as they are implemented in a clinical development environment. The following sections discuss research design and logistical factors that should be considered in this context.

Patient stratification: clarity of definitions

In order to discover biomarkers that accurately predict treatment outcome, researchers must first establish how response and non-response will be defined. At first glance this may seem simple enough since such definitions are a fundamental part of clinical research. However, response criteria for drug trials may differ from those required to identify individuals who are prone to response and the issue therefore deserves some attention. Indeed, in most disease states, established definitions of response involve arbitrary divisions within a wide range of patient outcomes.

In MDD for example, response in clinical trials is often defined as a 50% drop in scores on the Hamilton Depression Rating Scale (HAMD). However, a researcher using this criterion to stratify study populations might compare a "responder" whose HAMD dropped from 20 to 10 to a "non-responder" whose HAMD dropped from 20 to 11. Since it is unlikely that markers sensitive to a one-point difference on the HAMD would have much clinical relevance it is clear that response criteria used to assess treatment response across a population can be too arbitrary for the purposes of biomarker research.

The most obvious way to address this is to use more narrowly defined response and non-response criteria. For example, one might compare patients showing a high degree of response (e.g. using an established definition of remission) vs. those showing little or no response, while excluding patients showing partial response from the analysis. However, such approaches will significantly reduce the number of patients available for biomarker studies, which will have implications for the ability to adequately power the research (see below).

Another important consideration in stratifying patient populations is that in most CNS drug trials, placebo response will be indistinguishable from drug response. Consequently, a portion of "responders" will not have responded to the drug per se and will therefore contribute noise to any biomarker research in which they are included. Unfortunately, placebo response is a ubiquitous issue in clinical research and in many cases there may be little the biomarker researcher can do to address this issue other than to include sufficient numbers of patients to ensure as much as possible that true drug responders are fully represented in the test population. For some diseases, however, there are study designs that may be better suited to teasing drug response apart from placebo response. An example of this may be found in "randomized discontinuation" designs, in which patients who respond while under open-label drug treatment are randomly assigned to either remain on drug or receive placebo, with a primary endpoint of relapse within a given timeframe. This design does not entirely eliminate placebo effects, but it can reduce their impact, particularly since the long duration of such studies will tend to eliminate transient placebo effects and give a better picture of long-term outcomes.

Another consideration is that the measures used in clinical trials are often only moderately sensitive to drug-induced change. Indeed, many of the endpoints that are desirable from the perspective of a regulatory body in their evaluation of a drug's effects are much less well-suited to the stratification of patients for biomarker studies. The gold standard tools for assessing neurodegenerative diseases such as Alzheimer's and Parkinson's disease (i.e. the ADAS-COG and UPDRS), for example, are used because they are designed to assess the functional and behavioral impact of neurodegeneration. Assessments of the degree of brain damage using imaging techniques on the other hand have been shown to have only a poor relationship with functional or behavioral outcome variables. Similarly, cognitive batteries have been shown to be extremely sensitive in assessing disease progression, but unless the functional impact of changes in these measures can be established they cannot be used as primary endpoints. Nevertheless, biomarkers that are highly sensitive to changes in the underlying disease process (such as sophisticated imaging techniques or cognitive batteries) might be extremely useful in predicting drug efficacy or for stratification of disease populations, despite their limitations as primary endpoints. In such cases it will be essential that their inclusion in clinical trials is considered by drug developers at the earliest stages of the planning process.

Powering biomarker discovery

Given the modest number of subjects that are typically enrolled in Phase II programs and the need to further stratify these populations according to response or other factors, powering biomarker research studies will inevitably be an issue. Obviously, the expected effect size and standard deviation of the performance of the biomarkers will drive power calculations, but there are other important factors that must also be considered in determining how many patient samples should be included in research of this kind.

Increasing the number of patients included in clinical discovery research will increase the reliability of the findings. However, adding patients to clinical trials will have significant cost implications. Even if budget issues can be addressed there are practical limitations to how many patients can be screened using available biomarker discovery techniques. For example, due to the extreme complexity and large dynamic range of proteins found in blood, available proteomic discovery methods require the fractionation of a given blood sample into as many as 100 fractions. Since each fraction requires a separate mass spectrometry run, the analysis of even modest numbers of patients can involve years of machine time. That is, even if sufficient patient numbers are available to adequately power a biomarker discovery program, the logistics involved with so-called "unbiased" discovery methods will limit what can realistically be accomplished.

Nevertheless, the goal of discovery research is not to provide definitive answers, but rather to generate hypotheses which can subsequently be confirmed in well-controlled studies. Some researchers choose to accept the limitations of small pilot studies in hopes of identifying previously unknown putative markers that appear to be altered in response to a drug. If there are adequate time and resources to complete the discovery, confirmatory, and validation phases required to demonstrate the utility of these novel markers, then inclusion of an unbiased discovery phase has the potential to add significant value to a drug program. Unfortunately, time and resources are often in short supply in drug development.

Irrespective of whether the companion biomarker studies utilize discovery methodologies or a more targeted approach, a successful biomarker ultimately must meet disease-specific requirements for both sensitivity (the proportion of patients correctly identified by the test) and specificity (the proportion of patients correctly excluded by the test). Sensitivity will need to be high for markers of response since they will ultimately be used to identify which patients should receive the test drug: the standard of evidence required is essentially that of any regulatory-approved diagnostic or prognostic tool. Validation of such a tool will require substantial numbers of patients in order to provide regulators with compelling evidence that a representative patient sample has been tested.

On the other hand, markers of non-response are used to enrich clinical trial populations by excluding some of those who are unlikely to respond, which has far more limited regulatory and drug labeling implications and more flexibility as to the degree of specificity required. Fewer subjects will be required to achieve these aims since the consequence of reduced specificity is that some patients will be excluded from clinical trials that could have been included; while not ideal in that patient recruitment will be slowed, it is unlikely that their exclusion will negatively impact the ability to interpret the results from the study. The sensitivity and specificity requirements will therefore directly impact the number of subjects required and drug developers will need to carefully think through their requirements in the early stages of their planning.

Specimen collection and storage issues

Once the target population has been identified, decisions need to be made regarding the type of specimen that should be collected as well as the standard operating procedures (SOPs) for their collection. Although tissues derived from the disease site are ideal for biomarker research, they are not accessible within the context of most CNS clinical trials. Blood and urine, however, are collected routinely by all clinical research centers and can be excellent matrices for the conduct of many kinds of CNS biomarker research.

Unfortunately, the specimen collection methods used by most clinical sites (e.g. for routine clinical chemistry) are suboptimal for biomarker research. For example, delays in sample processing (i.e. latency to centrifugation or freezing) can significantly alter the amount and quality of a given protein in a specimen (Flower et al., 2000). Furthermore, latency to processing and other details related to clinical specimen handling are not routinely recorded by study staff. Indeed, hospital central laboratories are often ill-prepared to manage study-specific processing requirements and will batch samples for processing, which will by definition result in variability in processing latencies. Given that the changes in protein levels that can occur with these delays are as large as the anticipated effect size, this is a very significant issue. Fortunately, there is some evidence that keeping blood specimens on ice (a routine practice in many clinical trials if not clinical practice) will preserve at least some proteins that are affected by these issues. Still, even this is an imperfect solution since some proteins are temperature-sensitive. In any case, industry-sponsored clinical trials involve a great deal more scrutiny and methodological rigor than is possible in most academic research settings, and therefore are an excellent opportunity to collect high-quality specimens in an appropriately controlled environment.

The media into which specimens are collected can also have tremendous impact on the type of research that can be conducted. Blood tubes specifically designed for the purposes of genomics research (e.g. PAXgene tubes for DNA and RNA) are now in routine use. For proteomics research the picture is somewhat less clear due to the impact of collection tube type on protein content. Not only will the concentration of some proteins be different in plasma than serum (Findeisen *et al.*, 2005), but plasma collected in EDTA, sodium citrate, or heparin tubes will also each show different concentrations of certain proteins (Flower *et al.*, 2000).

Furthermore, each blood tube manufacturer issues its own recommendations for centrifugation speed and duration based on methods that produce optimal results, yet different centrifuge rotors are required to generate the required speeds for each tube type. Most clinics will not have access to multiple centrifuges or rotors and therefore the manufacturer's recommendations will be ignored at least some of the time. Providing research sites with centrifuges (preferably refrigerated) is one possible solution, but in any case the scrutiny applied to sample processing parameters will need to increase if such variables are to be controlled.

These issues speak to a more fundamental problem in specimen collection: the lack of accepted and broadly implemented SOPs. The SOPs employed within most research sites were developed internally, leading to idiosyncratic approaches to specimen collection. While universal SOPs may be difficult to implement within existing hospital or clinic central laboratory processes, they are the only way to ensure that the quality of specimens is adequate to the complexity of the task. Several initiatives to create appropriate standards and best practices are under way (e.g. within the Human Proteome Organization; Rai *et al.*, 2005), but it will be critical that these initiatives are truly data-driven and that buy-in is sought from numerous medical sources if they are to be broadly implemented. In any case, since the impact of sample handling varies from protein to protein, the only way to be certain that optimal sample handling methods are developed is to systematically assess sample handling effects on every protein that might be of medical interest. Obviously this lies outside what is currently feasible, but it illustrates the direction in which the field ultimately needs to move.

Long-term storage of biospecimens is another important consideration that is often overlooked. When specimens are collected it is ideal if they are divided into aliquots of an appropriate volume for the purposes of the research to which they will be applied. The optimal aliquot size will vary with the technology, but since they may be needed for multiple studies and no more than two freeze/thaw cycles should be allowed if at all possible (Mitchell *et al.*, 2005), then smaller aliquots are more desirable than large aliquots. For example, a 10 ml blood tube will yield about 3 ml of plasma, which will in turn yield approximately 6×500 µl aliquots. This is a reasonable number of aliquots since each one is large enough for most kinds of biomarker research and one blood draw will support up to six studies. Smaller aliquots may also make sense for some kinds of research, but each aliquot will take up a "slot" within the long-term storage freezer and so doubling the number of aliquots will double the cost for storage.

The temperature at which samples are kept is another consideration. Long-term storage of specimens in liquid nitrogen is probably the most cost-effective and efficient method, though mechanical ($-80°$C) freezers can also be used. In either case, systems for temperature monitoring and to manage catastrophic events are not just good laboratory practice requirements, but are simply good sense for such irreplaceable materials.

Selection of omics approach

Before a clinical trial program begins, drug developers should design the key elements of their companion biomarker program. This is important since the type of specimens and other data that need to be collected within the clinical trials will vary from one approach to another. Since many clinical trials will require years to complete the activities between design and database lock it is likely that the methods available during the design phase will have improved by the time biomarker analysis begins. Although this may limit to some degree the types of decisions that can be made, even basic up-front decisions such as whether DNA, RNA, or protein will be studied will be useful through enabling effective and appropriate specimen collection. On the other hand, drug developers may wish to accelerate the completion of a biomarker program by conducting analyses as soon as specimens are collected during the trial. This will force detailed methodological decisions to be made in the earliest phases of the program.

Irrespective of which methods are selected, some common issues will need to be addressed in relation to how these choices impact the design of the clinical trials. Currently available "unbiased" biomarker discovery technologies such as gene microarray, copy number variant (CNV), and proteomic discovery methodologies are well-suited to generating hypotheses, but subsequent validation is critical given the high false-positive discovery rate and very large, complex data sets. Furthermore, these discovery technologies are ill-suited to high-throughput validation studies or use in clinical settings; any discoveries made using these techniques will require several subsequent stages of research using robust quantitative technologies. For the foreseeable future, therefore, the use of undirected biomarker discovery approaches will usually be impractical in the context of stratifying patients on the basis of treatment outcome for the simple reason that they will take too long to implement.

However, these discovery technologies may be well suited to guiding future biomarker studies if applied during the earliest stages of drug development. Unbiased discovery work can, for example, be conducted in cell lines and animal models using pooled samples, a cost- and time-saving approach that is less practical for human research due to inter-individual variability. Basic research of this kind can give researchers valuable information about drug-induced changes that may not be obvious based on current knowledge, further informing subsequent directed research efforts during clinical development. Similarly, discovery methods can be applied to specimens collected during Phase I. Such techniques could be ideally suited to identifying previously unknown pharmacodynamic markers (i.e. markers whose presence is altered in response to dose and pharmacokinetic changes), which can prove extremely useful in subsequent studies.

In addition to so-called unbiased approaches, omics technologies have advanced to the degree that more targeted discovery approaches are both practical and cost-effective. For most diseases there is a large and growing list of putative markers that have been associated with disease progression, relevant biological systems, or even drug response, which can inform these more directed approaches to response biomarker discovery. Modern quantitative proteomic (e.g. multiple reaction monitoring mass spectrometry) and genomic (e.g. quantitative single nucleotide polymorphisms – SNPs) technologies are now sufficiently high-throughput and reliable that they can be used to systematically screen hundreds or even thousands of potentially important targets in relation to patient outcomes. As these technologies improve – and knowledge regarding relevant biological systems improves – the application of such "biomarker batteries" has the potential to enable discovery and preliminary validation of drug response markers within timelines acceptable to commercial drug development, while eliminating much of the uncertainty associated with conventional "unbiased" discovery methods.

The one key drawback to this approach is that biomarker batteries rely upon the knowledge that is available at the time of their implementation, which is at best incomplete and at worst misleading. Furthermore, the factors that alter individual response may not be related to known disease-related systems. Nevertheless, systematic testing of previously identified markers seems an obvious place to start, particularly given that the performance of a given marker, when combined with other markers, may be much better than when assessed in isolation.

Another important consideration in selecting which technology to employ relates to how easily the technologies could be implemented in the clinic. Biomarker measurement technologies such as MRM MS have not yet been used in support of regulatory approvals (other than in the context of measuring small molecules) and therefore will face a series of regulatory hurdles before they can be utilized in all phases of drug development. Furthermore, a high degree of expertise is required for the implementation of many biomarker research methods, making them impractical for broad implementation. Even well-developed technologies should be carefully evaluated in terms of the goals of the program. For example, immunoassays have been successfully used, but unless high-quality antibodies are available will themselves require significant and risky further development activities.

All biomarker research technologies are comparatively new and, as with all new technologies, may lack the reliability one generally requires for regulatory-compliant research. However, the power and potential of these technologies are undeniable and their routine use in drug development is therefore inevitable. Irrespective of the approach or methodology, though, early integration into drug development and proper planning and design (see Figure 3) will be essential if the potential is to be realized.

Marker panels: when one is not enough

The mapping of the human genome has led to an explosion in research and understanding in virtually every aspect of medicine, yet this increased understanding has itself revealed new layers of complexity and heterogeneity in human disease. Huntington's disease (HD), for example, is caused by a single gene expansion on chromosome 4, yet latency to symptom onset, speed of progression, and symptom manifestation all vary widely across this population. That is, even in the extreme case where a single gene mutation is clearly causal in a given disease, the mutation by itself does not explain many aspects of the disease that are clearly relevant to treatment, outcome, and the quality of a patient's life. Other variables and techniques must be explored to address this variability, including epigenetic phenomena, proteomics, metabolomics, imaging, and the use of more sophisticated clinical assessment tools.

One method to address this variability is to combine multiple markers into a single panel for use as a diagnostic or prognostic test. The Mammaprint and Oncotype DX gene-based tests in breast cancer and the OVA1 protein-based test in ovarian cancer are early FDA-approved examples of this approach. These marker panels utilize algorithms to assemble data from multiple markers into a single score that can be used to make clinical decisions. The success of this approach is undeniable; however, it is not without its challenges.

First, many of the markers that one might contemplate incorporating into a panel will have previously been patented for use in diagnosing the diseases in question. While this has

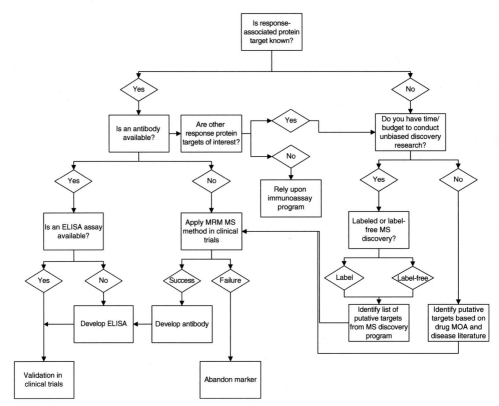

Figure 3. Example decision tree for planning a proteomics-based biomarker companion research program.

the potential to create a murky intellectual property environment, there are several ways to address the issue. For example, such patents do not prevent innovators from seeking protection for a specific combination of markers as classifiers, provided they can demonstrate that the patented markers do not by themselves produce as favorable sensitivity and specificity as was seen with the panel.

Second, there is the enormous computational complexity in identifying optimal combinations of markers (see discussion below) which will impact the likelihood of a successful outcome. In some respects this creates an opportunity, however, since proprietary algorithms can not only solve this problem, but can provide innovators with an avenue for intellectual property protection and commercial benefit, as was accomplished with the Oncotype DX test.

Third, if a marker panel is to be used to select patients for treatment it will be essential that the panel can be broadly implemented in clinical settings. If clinicians must undergo a lengthy or convoluted process for acquiring test results then the uptake of both the test and drug may be suboptimal. Since complex multiplexed tests may be difficult to implement outside state-of-the-art laboratory facilities a test optimization program should be incorporated into the development process, adding time and regulatory complexity.

These are all manageable challenges, but if appropriate planning is not undertaken as early as possible in the process then significant delay will be inevitable to the drug development program in which such panels are to be incorporated.

Analysis of complex data sets

Biomarker methodologies produce a great deal of complex data. Sequencing a single human genome, for example, can produce up to 30 terabytes of raw data. Given that the "1000 dollar genome" target is expected to be met within the next few years, the requirements for biomarker data storage can only be expected to grow. Yet the storage issues are minor in comparison to the challenges associated with analyzing such enormous data sets.

Seeking optimal combinations of markers to serve as classifiers in relation to treatment outcome is an excellent illustration of the challenge. If one were to investigate every possible combination of markers, and given n observations, then the number of marker panels that must be evaluated is 2^n. When small numbers of markers are investigated this approach is ideal since eventually the best fit to the data will be identified. However, the exponential requirements for analysis means that only a small number of markers can be added to the equation before the processing requirements exceed the capabilities of available supercomputing platforms. Until the day when such calculations are feasible, bioinformaticians must employ algorithms that narrow down the number of calculations to a more manageable subset. The problem with such approaches, however, is that different algorithms tend to produce different results. The onus will be on the developer to convince the regulatory bodies of the utility of the algorithm they have chosen.

Another key issue in the analysis of biomarker data is that the questions are becoming increasingly complex. A critical example of this lies in the observation that many seemingly unrelated diseases share common mechanisms. Ulcers are now known to be primarily caused by *H. pylori* infections. Inflammation appears to play a key role in numerous diseases including heart disease, many types of cancer, Alzheimer's disease, and many others. Similarly, insulin-related growth factor is associated with many conditions, ranging from growth disorders such as Laron's syndrome, to aging-related diseases such as diabetes and cancer. Historically, these relationships were often discovered by serendipity, but there are a growing number of successful examples of systematic investigations into these underlying mechanisms. However, at present there is only limited availability of computing platforms capable of securely accessing, storing, and analyzing the complex clinical, demographic, and biomarker data that will enable such research.

As medical practice moves toward comprehensive electronic data records many of these challenges will be addressed, assuming that obvious ethical issues related to anonymization and access to confidential health records can be overcome. Nevertheless, while clinical data sets tend to be small in relation to genomic, proteomic, and imaging data sets, they are complex in their own right given the use of multiple data formats, adverse event coding conventions, language translation issues, and so on. Common data format is also an issue for the biomarker technologies since even within a given technique the equipment manufacturers tend to utilize idiosyncratic data formats and outputs, complicating the aggregation of data across platforms.

These are not trivial challenges. Given the cost and complexity of constructing regulatory-compliant supercomputing facilities, as well as the highly specialized expertise required to analyze the data generated from clinical biomarker research, the most logical solution lies with centralized hubs of computing hardware, software, and specialized expertise. Numerous centralized platforms have been built to address some of these needs, but these efforts will need to expand substantially if they are to service the broader academic and industry research communities.

Other approaches: retrospective analysis of biomarker data from Phases II and III: drug rescue

Although regulatory bodies have had relatively few test cases of drug/biomarker co-development approvals, the recent (July 17, 2009) FDA-approved label changes for cetuximab and panitumumab in the treatment of colorectal cancer in patients with wild-type KRAS status has established precedent for the use of *retrospective* biomarker data to identify responsive populations. AstraZeneca was similarly able to receive marketing authorization for gefitinib from EMEA on July 1, 2009 based on the evaluation of patient subgroup response in their Phase III trials.

While these were no doubt special cases, these approvals illustrate the potential to utilize similar techniques to conduct retrospective "drug rescue" programs in which responsive subpopulations are used not just to optimize treatment, but to secure approval of an effective medication when it would otherwise have failed during development. Even in the likely event that most of these programs will require at least one additional positive Phase III pivotal trial, the relatively modest additional investment this would require (in comparison to the total cost of development to that point) makes this an attractive proposition.

Numerous companies are now pursuing such approaches to drug repositioning, and as the methodologies evolve, biomarker-based drug rescue will likely become an important failsafe for drug developers. However, this underscores the importance of collecting high-quality specimens during clinical trials, even if the need for these collections is hypothetical. Indeed, as discussed above, for such collection efforts to be useful it is critical that specimen collection parameters, biomarker research technologies and various study design issues be carefully thought through prior to the initiation of clinical trials.

Regulatory issues

The patient populations described in a drug label will be defined by the patient populations included in Phase III. In other words, if a given panel of genes is used to define this population then appropriately developed clinical tests for this same panel of genes must be available in time for the launch of the drug. The need to undertake simultaneous regulatory approval processes for both drug and biomarker adds significant complexity to the development process. It is also an inevitable consequence of personalized medicine since the regulatory bodies will have limited freedom to make such a process easier. Indeed, as diseases themselves become increasingly defined by their underlying biochemistry it is likely that the regulators will take more interest, not less, in the standard of evidence required to define treatment populations.

Unfortunately, the regulatory guidances to industry in this field are to date of limited assistance since they primarily address markers identified prior to the initiation of clinical trials and therefore represent a special – and comparatively simple – example of biomarker research. Nevertheless, the need for clarification and expansion of these guidances has been a major topic of discussion within the FDA and EMEA and at time of writing new guidances were being considered. However, waiting for such guidance is not a practical option for most developers and there is certainly no guarantee they will be a panacea. Innovative approaches must be considered and implemented.

Most pharmaceutical companies have limited experience in the regulatory challenges associated with diagnostic and prognostic marker approval processes. While this is changing, many pharma and biotech companies rely on partnering to meet their companion diagnostic development needs, adding yet another layer of complexity to the process. Still, these challenges are manageable provided appropriate processes and infrastructure are in place, appropriate planning occurs far enough in advance, and biomarker research activities are fully integrated with the drug development process.

Ethical issues

When designing informed consent forms (ICFs) for clinical trials it is essential that appropriate wording be included to deal with issues specific to biomarker research. All too often informed consent forms describe very specific studies that were conceived before the clinical program began, but which require modification years later when the study is complete. Technologies and methods may evolve during the conduct of a clinical trial that might more appropriately address drug development questions, but if consents are overly rigid researchers will lack the flexibility they require to implement such methods. Furthermore, specimens collected in rigorously controlled clinical trials are extremely valuable, yet only a small portion of the collected specimens are required for most kinds of biomarker research. If ICFs do not specifically allow for additional research to be conducted then valuable research materials will be wasted. While re-consenting patients may theoretically be possible, it is impractical in most cases. It is critical therefore to work with regulators and ethics committees to devise ICF wording that protects and informs the patient, while ensuring that important research avenues remain open.

A core ethical issue in clinical research is the importance of maintaining the anonymity of the patient. Historically, this was a relatively simple issue to address: patient numbers are assigned to separate patient data from patient medical records. However, advances in medical technology have introduced a significant new wrinkle to this: it is currently impossible to anonymize a whole genome sequence. Brain images and even unique protein, CNV, or SNP signatures may well have the same problem. Given the power and potential of these technologies it is inconceivable that any rational legislation would exclude their collection. However, the methods and platforms used to collect and analyze such data will likely need to evolve in order to address very legitimate ethical concerns regarding patient privacy.

One possible solution would be the creation of "data fortresses" whereby sensitive patient data could be independently managed, analyzed, and stored but which could not be accessed by unauthorized individuals. The secure data tunnels, storage platforms, and regulatory-compliant facilities seen in most industry data centers could provide a model for such data fortresses, but few of the supercomputing facilities involved with high-end biomarker research are currently capable of meeting such requirements. Nevertheless, unless the anonymity of the patient can be maintained the ethical issues will remain and therefore solutions will need to be found.

The end game: validation

Once a classifier of drug response has been identified from data collected in Phase II, it must be validated in sufficient numbers of patients to be representative of a real-world population. Unfortunately, appropriate validation populations can only be accessed through the conduct of additional clinical trials, which will in most cases be pivotal trials in Phase III. This introduces a number of important considerations for the drug developer.

One such consideration relates to how to most effectively undertake validation within Phase III. If the treatment population is defined using a biomarker identified using a relatively small number of subjects from Phase II, then there is a very real possibility that the findings will not be replicated and Phase III outcomes will be compromised. On the other hand, if analyses using the biomarker-defined population are only undertaken as secondary endpoints, then the results will have limited utility in the drug approval process should the drug fail in the broader population.

It is highly desirable therefore for developers to have as much confidence as possible in the utility of their response classifiers from data derived in Phase II or other sources. This requires at least some degree of validation to occur during these phases, which is challenging given the small sample sizes. When limited patient samples are available a typical approach is to divide the population into a "training" set, for the purposes of discovery, and a "test" set which is used for validation, which of course further divides a sample that is already small.

Although the training and test approach is a common and accepted approach, it is not necessarily the most robust use of the data. For example, an n-fold approach (Simon, 2008) identifies then validates classifiers using n different divisions of the same sample set rather than the single division used in a training and test approach. If the same classifier is seen repeatedly then confidence in its utility will be increased. While the acceptance of such approaches is by no means universal, they are theoretically more robust and powerful than more traditional approaches.

Another way to address the issue of using non-validated markers to define Phase III populations may lie in the use of various novel statistical approaches in defining primary endpoints. For example, conventional Phase III inclusion/exclusion criteria and endpoints might be employed, but in studies powered in such a way as to conduct a separate planned analysis using the subset of these patients identified by the marker. There are sample size adjustments available to allow for such dual-endpoint approaches and provided agreement can be reached with the regulatory bodies as to the appropriateness of such a method, they could effectively be used by drug developers to hedge their bets while increasing the likelihood that an optimal patient population will be identified for receiving the treatment. Indeed, approaches such as this may be essential in order to encourage drug developers to take the risk of defining their populations in this manner.

Summary: personalized medicines and biomarkers in Phase II

Personalized medicine is already having a tremendous impact on medical practice and its importance will continue to grow. Biomarker technologies have proven their mettle in a number of applications and practical methods are now available that enable their inclusion in the drug development process. Nevertheless, many challenges must be overcome before their use can become truly widespread in Phase II. For drug developers, methodical planning and centralization of resources as well as research standards and best practices will be critical to achieving the huge potential of this field. CNS drug developers and their development plans will need to adapt to incorporate the changes brought by personalized medicines.

References

Chapel, S., Hutmacher, M. M., Haig, G., et al. (2009). Exposure-response analysis in patients with schizophrenia to assess the effect of asenapine on QTc prolongation. J Clin Pharmacol, 49, 1297–308.

Cutler, N. R. (2001). Pharmacokinetics studies of antipsychotics in healthy volunteers versus patients. J Clin Psychiat, 62[suppl 5], 10–13.

Cutler, N. R. and Sramek, J. J. (2000). Investigator perspective on MTD: practical application of an MTD definition—has it accelerated development? *J Clin Pharmacol*, 40, 1184–7.

Dimond, K. R., Pande, A. C., Lamoreaux, L., and Pierce, M. W. (1996). Effect of gabapentin (Neurontin) on mood and well-being in patients with epilepsy. *Prog Neuropsychopharmacol Biol Psychiat*, 20, 407–17.

Feltner, D. E., Hill, C., Lenderking, W., Williams, V., and Morlock, R. (2009). Development of a patient-reported assessment to identify placebo responders in a generalized anxiety disorder trial. *J Psychiat Res*, 43, 1223–30.

Findeisen, P., Sismanidis, D., Riedl, M., Costina, V., and Neumaier, M. (2005). Preanalytical impact of sample handling on proteome profiling experiments with matrix-assisted laser desorption/ionization time-of-flight mass spectrometry. *Clin Chem*, 51, 2409–11.

Flower, L., Ahuja, R. H., Humphries, S. E., and Mohamed-Ali, V. (2000). Effects of sample handling on the stability of interleukin 6, tumour necrosis factor and leptin. *Cytokine*, 12, 1712–16.

Frueh, F. W., Amur, S., Mummaneni, P., *et al.* (2008). Pharmacogenomic biomarker information in drug labels approved by the United States food and drug administration: prevalence of related drug use. *Pharmacotherapy*, 28, 992–8.

Grimwood, S. and Hartig, P. R. (2009). Target site occupancy: Emerging generalizations from clinical and preclinical studies. *Pharmacol Therapeut*, 122, 281–301.

Huezo-Diaz, P., Uher, R., Smith, R., *et al.* (2009). Moderation of antidepressant response by the serotonin transporter gene. *Brit J Psychiatr*, 195, 30–8.

Keller, M., Montgomery, S., Ball, W., *et al.* (2006). Lack of efficacy of the substance P (neurokinin1 receptor) antagonist aprepitant in the treatment of major depressive disorder. *Biol Psychiat*, 59, 216–23.

Kemeny, M. E., Rosenwasser, L. J., Panettieri, R. A., *et al.* (2007). Placebo response in asthma: A robust and objective phenomenon. *J Allergy Clin Immunol*, 119, 1375–81.

Killackey, E. and Yung, A. R. (2007). Effectiveness of early intervention in psychosis. *Curr Opin Psychiat*, 20, 121–5.

Kim, H., Lim, S.-W., *et al.* (2006). Monoamine transporter gene polymorphisms and antidepressant response in Koreans with late-life depression. *J Am Med Assoc*, 296, 1609–18.

Krams, M., Lees, K. R., Hacke, W., *et al.* (2003). Acute stroke therapy by inhibition of neutrophils (ASTIN): an adaptive dose-response study of UK-279,276 in acute ischemic stroke. *Stroke*, 34, 2543–8.

Lalonde, R. L., Kowalski, K. G., Hutmacher, M. M., *et al.* (2007). Model-based drug development. *Clin Pharmacol Therapeut*, 82, 21–32.

Mitchell, B. L., Yasuie, Y., Lia, C. I., Fitzpatrick, A. L., and Lampea, P. D. (2005). Impact of freeze-thaw cycles and storage time on plasma samples used in mass spectrometry based biomarker discovery projects. *Cancer Informatics*, 1, 98–104.

Ouellet, D., Werth, J., Parekh, N., *et al.* (2009). The use of a clinical utility index to compare insomnia compounds: a quantitative basis for benefit risk assessment. *Clin Pharmacol Therapeut*, 85 (3), 277–82.

Rai, A. J., Gelfand, C. A., Haywood, B., *et al.* (2005). HUPO Plasma Proteome Project specimen collection and handling: towards the standardization of parameters for plasma proteome samples. *Proteomics*, 5, 3262–77.

Simon, R. (2008). Designs and adaptive analysis plans for pivotal clinical trials of therapeutics and companion diagnostics. *Expert Opin Med Diagnostics*, 2, 721–29.

Sinyor, M., Levitt, A. J., Cheung, A. H., *et al.* (2010). Does inclusion of a placebo arm influence response to active antidepressant treatment in randomized controlled trials? Results from pooled and meta-analyses. *J Clin Psychiat*, 71 (3), 270–79.

Slamon, D. J., Leyland-Jones, B., Shak, S., *et al.* (2001). Use of chemotherapy plus a monoclonal antibody against HER2 for metastatic breast cancer that overexpresses HER2. *New Engl J Med*, 344, 783–92.

CNS drug development – Phase III

Judith Dunn, Penny Randall, and Amir Kalali

A mission defined by multiple stakeholders

The goal of a Phase III or late-stage development program is to generate an extensive, clinical dataset sufficient to achieve authorization/approval from global health authorities to market the drug, ensure access to the drug from pricing and reimbursement groups, and facilitate uptake of the medication by physicians and patients. The required evidence must, at a minimum, define the appropriate populations for use, provide pharmacokinetic/ pharmacodynamic-based dosing instructions, clearly delineate the safety and tolerability profiles, demonstrate clinical utility that outweighs identified risks, and articulate the economic benefit associated with use of the new agent versus available therapies.

Although in general each stakeholder has a requirement for evidence of safety and overall benefit, the specific type of data considered relevant and compelling by each decision-maker varies. For example, an antidepressant drug can achieve regulatory approval on the basis of a 2–3 point mean difference between drug and placebo on the Hamilton Depression Rating Scale. Few physicians utilize this psychometric instrument in daily practice. In order to prescribe and use a new antidepressant, doctors and their patients require additional measures of efficacy whose clinical relevance is more easily understood at the individual level versus the statistical significance of mean change in a population. Finally, although payers accept conventional regulatory endpoints as proof of efficacy, satisfactory reimbursement requires evidence of benefit beyond the current standard of care, which often can necessitate the inclusion of yet another measurement of efficacy in the development program. It quickly becomes apparent that the requirement to provide convincing data to a variety of stakeholders adds time, cost, and complexity to late-stage development programs. Such complexity burdens the clinical trial investigators and participating subjects, and may contribute to increasing failure rates. This is particularly true in CNS disorders, where many endpoints are subjective and the outcomes can be influenced by the measures themselves.

Between 2007 and 2010 there were 83 late-stage development failures, 18% of which were compounds being studied in CNS indications (Arrowsmith, 2011). The majority of these compounds (66%) failed to demonstrate efficacy. There are two obvious areas of focus when hypothesizing the reasons for late-stage efficacy failure; the molecules themselves and the methodology.

Phase III development of a drug candidate is initiated following an average of 5.5 years of discovery/pre-clinical validation efforts and 4 years of early clinical investigation

Essential CNS Drug Development, ed. A. Kalali, Sheldon Preskorn, J. Kwentus, and Stephen M. Stahl. Published by Cambridge University Press. © Cambridge University Press 2012.

(Paul *et al.*, 2010). During the decade of research leading to Phase III, the relevance of the molecular target to the disease state is validated using in vitro and translational approaches; penetration of the molecule into the CNS is confirmed via imaging and CSF sampling; the safety profile is established to be appropriate for continued human investigation in Phase I studies; and the efficacy of the molecule in addressing symptoms or disease progression in the population of interest is demonstrated by means of Proof of Concept study (or studies). Therefore, once the decision to move a compound to Phase III is taken, if the early development process was effective, the viability of the molecule as an efficacious agent should not be in dispute. Arguably, clinical trial methodology is the major determinant of demonstration of efficacy in CNS Phase III trials.

The demand for innovative medications addressing unmet clinical need requires novel mechanisms engaging novel targets. Phase III clinical trial methodology must keep pace with the evolving biology to maximize efficacy signal detection in new clinical domains and support cost-effective development programs which more consistently result in new marketed medications.

Study populations

There is increasing disparity between the group of clinical trial subjects considered of interest to physicians and payers versus those that sponsors feel best enable delineation of safety and efficacy profiles. This is especially true when studying molecules with novel mechanisms of action, where available information regarding safety and efficacy may be limited to the Phase I and II populations.

From a sponsor perspective, inclusion/exclusion criteria must be specifically designed to ensure that the resulting safety and efficacy data are interpretable and support global registration. In the 1993 "Guideline for the Study and Evaluation of Gender Differences in Clinical Evaluation of Drugs", the FDA stated that drugs should be studied prior to approval in subjects representing a full range of patients likely to receive the drug once it is marketed. Based on this guidance, in order to obtain marketing authorization, sponsors are required to understand differences in dose-response, effect size, and tolerability in a variety of demographic (age, gender, race) groups and other subsets of the population (e.g. renally or hepatically impaired).

Because such population heterogeneity can impact treatment effect, the early development program should include elements (e.g. in vitro studies, exposure in special populations, PKPD modeling) which de-risk inclusion of population heterogeneity in Phase III. Additionally, prospectively defined statistical methodology such as adaptation and stratification should be considered in the Phase III program to enhance understanding of efficacy and safety signals in diverse populations while providing the drug the best chance to demonstrate efficacy. Finally, special populations such as renally impaired subjects should be studied outside the pivotal trials primarily designated to support registration; questions regarding safety and efficacy should be examined in smaller trials containing more extensive measures of exposure and tolerability.

Despite regulatory requirements for diversity, physicians and payers increasingly argue that Phase III inclusion and exclusion criteria identify a group of patients not representative of the population to whom the medication will be prescribed. For example, the NIMH sponsored Sequenced Treatment Alternatives to Relieve Depression (STAR*D) project used very broad inclusion criteria to examine the efficacy of medications used to treat Major

Depressive Disorder (Rush *et al.*, 2006a, 2006b). It has been suggested that less than 25% of depressed subjects enrolled in this highly inclusive trial would meet typical entry criteria for Phase III clinical trials (Wisniewski *et al.*, 2009).

Perhaps contributing to the perception of insufficient generalizability of Phase III trial results is the fact that although regulators provide specific guidance regarding demographic diversity, there is little guidance addressing symptom heterogeneity. Health authorities world-wide have traditionally relied on clinical diagnostic/classification methods (DSM, ICD) to broadly define populations appropriate for inclusion in clinical trials. With such broad clinical criteria, it is possible for subjects to meet the clinical diagnosis for the disease under study, while failing to exhibit the symptoms which the compound targets. To ensure that new, highly specific mechanisms of action are studied in patients who can realize the most benefit, inclusion/exclusion criteria should be utilized to identify patient populations within particular disorders who exhibit the target symptoms for which the drug is designed. The deliberate selection of patients exhibiting relevant symptoms (and therefore most likely to best respond) is an appropriate method of enhancing signal detection. Improved signal detection reduces the number of subjects required to meet statistical criteria and improves success rate. Fewer failed trials in turn decreases the time and cost required to generate the two registration trials required for approval. The cost and time savings realized by appropriate patient selection allow developers to address external stakeholder (physician and patient) requirements to better understand the clinical utility of the compound in observational trials designed to establish clinical relevance and inform prescribing practices for broader populations versus meeting statistical significance. Such trials can be conducted within the Phase III development program to support the generation of a reasonably sized safety database to support approval as well as generate data to assist market access and educate physicians.

The strategy to run a few streamlined trials to demonstrate efficacy while generating additional safety and differentiation data in observational or "real-world" trials is not without risk. Drug developers must balance the increased likelihood of clinical success with the possibility that the populations used to demonstrate efficacy may be specifically indicated in labeling granted by health authorities, thereby limiting market access. There are several mechanisms in place (End of Phase II meetings, Scientific Advice and Special Protocol Assessments) for sponsors to offset this risk by providing a clinically sound rationale to support selection of a study population that will achieve the desired broad product labeling.

The ability of inclusion/exclusion criteria to identify a Phase III population with the appropriate clinical and demographic features is directly linked to adherence to these criteria. Confirmation of subject eligibility by a third party or technology is an increasingly popular method to ensure appropriate enrollment. A collaborative approach between investigators and outside reviewers is a reasonable and effective means of maximizing the benefit of well-designed selection criteria.

Comparators

In most therapeutic areas, clinical trial endpoints are quantitative and objective (e.g. laboratory testing, imaging technology). Psychiatric and several neurological disorders (e.g. pain), however, utilize subjective measures of effectiveness and reliable biomarkers or quantitative surrogate indicators of response have yet to be identified. Treatment response observed in subjective trials is related not only to the mechanism-derived benefit of the active medication but also to the psychosocial context in which it was delivered. Several factors related to patients, physicians, treatment environment, and their interactions contribute to the contextual component of this response (Colagiuri, 2010). The intended utility of a placebo comparator is to measure clinical response unrelated to active medication. Efficacy related to the drug under study is defined as the difference between the response to placebo and active drug. The use of placebo as comparator affords researchers the opportunity to achieve maximum treatment separation, which increases signal detection, maximizes statistical power, and decreases the number of subjects exposed to experimental compounds.

The response to placebo in psychiatric clinical trials is increasing over time, and is approaching 30% in several indications (Kinon et al., 2011; Walsh et al., 2002). This increased response dilutes the magnitude of the observed efficacy signal that can be attributed to drug, and thus is responsible for clinical trial failure. Several factors are hypothesized to contribute to this problem, including but not limited to incorrect diagnosis of trial participants, poor psychometric instruments, flawed assessments by investigators, high drop-out rates, and neurobiology. Remedial approaches receiving the most attention are improving rating accuracy via training, rating surveillance technology, blinding investigators to the start of active medication via blinded run-in periods, decreasing time spent in the physician office, and improving the sensitivity of the psychometric instruments used. Although much effort is being spent on reducing the impact of placebo response, no single method has been identified as significantly better than another. It is likely that a combination of features contribute to placebo response, and researchers should control as many of these features as possible without compromising the integrity of the trial.

The steadily increasing placebo response in psychiatry and neurology trials, debate regarding ethical justification of placebo, and requests from patients, clinicians, payers and some health authorities for comparative effectiveness data are leading to a steady increase in active-comparator studies. The comparator chosen is usually the Standard of Care or best available therapy. A trial of this type allows comparison of risk-benefit profiles between the two different therapies, which is of interest to several stakeholders, including physicians and payers. In addition, the use of an active comparator removes the ethical dilemma of placebo-controlled trials.

Despite the interest in comparative data, there are risks associated with a trial design of this type: the number of subjects required to show statistical superiority to active medication is large and will increase the duration and cost of the trial as well as increasing the risk that the medication under investigation will fail to demonstrate an efficacy advantage. Failure of a compound to demonstrate superiority in efficacy versus an active comparator may lead researchers to overlook other important differentiating features of the compound such as safety or tolerability advantages. As novel mechanisms of action increasingly target unmet medical needs, relevant comparators are often not available, and inappropriate comparison to active comparators may lead to incorrect decisions regarding the fate of the compound.

Placebo-controlled trials offer the best opportunity to demonstrate maximal efficacy with the fewest number of patients. Often, this choice of comparator is the most methodologically valid for supporting registration with global health authorities. However, researchers must ensure patients who receive placebo are not subject to serious risk or irreversible harm.

Comparative data, examining endpoints suspected to be differentiating, are likely best generated in observational trials specifically designed to demonstrate anticipated advantages without compromising the efficacy data generated in the pivotal trials.

Endpoints

The ideal design for a clinical trial includes a single primary endpoint that completely characterizes the disease under study and efficiently evaluates treatment efficacy (ICH Guideline, 1998). It is well accepted that these endpoints must be clinically meaningful, sensitive to change, and relatively simple to administer. The study of CNS disorders is complicated by the fact that disorders are characterized by broad groups of symptoms, and medications are likely to impact some, but not all, of these symptoms. Historically, health authorities have primarily focused on the direct impact of the medication on the disease under study to support labeled indications for alleviation of symptoms, disease modification, or relapse prevention. The vast majority of drugs in any CNS indication have been approved using the same primary efficacy variable (e.g. HAMD, HAMA, ADAS-Cog); endpoints designed and selected with the goal of demonstrating broad clinical benefit to obtain a labeled indication for the largest number of individuals possible.

More recently, however, the psychiatry community in particular has begun to realize that since the diagnostic criteria of most CNS disorders is a heterogeneous collection of symptoms which occur in varying proportions within disease populations, the maximum effect of a drug may not be recognized using these traditional, broad measures (Targum et al., 2008). Consequently, it is becoming more common for pharmaceutical companies to seek indications for specific symptoms within psychiatric disorders (e.g. negative symptoms in schizophrenia, irritability associated with autism) in order to best demonstrate the clinical utility of a drug's mechanism of action. The upside of this approach may be increased success in Phase III due to optimized clinical target selection.

Several trade-offs, however, accompany this strategy. The clinical relevance and risk/benefit profile of a targeted therapy will need to be demonstrated for regulators, as well as healthcare providers and consumers. In many cases such evidence will require the development of new efficacy measures, a lengthy and expensive undertaking that can require several years to accomplish. The planning and investment for alternative measures of efficacy must therefore begin, at some risk, as early as Phase I in a development program, prior to generation of a dataset supporting development of the molecule. In addition, an approval label resulting from a new, targeted efficacy measure will most likely be limited to the population studied, and will therefore have decreased market penetration and lower commercial value. Pharmaceutical companies have a complex value proposition to calculate when considering the development options for a new compound: (1) to make an early investment in a targeted outcome measure, which may have an increased chance of technical success but a decreased chance of regulatory success and lower commercial value; or (2) to conduct a traditional development plan, the endpoints of which will address broader clinical domains with endpoints traditionally accepted by regulators, but with a decreased likelihood of technical success due to the suboptimal coupling of pharmacology to clinic target(s). The combination of variables and their relative impact on decision-making is ultimately a balance of scientific and financial risk-taking, and varies between indications and companies, each of whom have a different tolerance for risk, requirement for success, and competing portfolio priorities.

In addition to the efficacy dataset utilized by health authorities to support approval and labeling, drug developers must also provide data which inform healthcare providers and consumers (physicians, patients, caregivers, and payers). These stakeholders are less interested in benefit versus placebo than in understanding comparative efficacy versus available therapies. Additionally, evaluation of clinical benefit relative to quality of life factors such as disease burden, independence, productivity, and adherence inform healthcare decisions, and are even more important when traditional efficacy measures show little benefit versus available therapy.

Patient-reported outcomes (PROs) are an effective means of demonstrating differentiation from the perspective of the patient or caregiver and have been successfully used to facilitate uptake of new drugs by patients, inform prescribers, and support reimbursement. Consistent with the practice of executing streamlined, uncomplicated pivotal trials to maximize the potential for technical success and support registration, PROs have traditionally been included in observational trials, or often even delayed until post-approval trials. Their utility has traditionally been realized in domains outside those labeled by regulators (e.g. dependency, treatment satisfaction, adherence). More recently, regulators have joined payers and other stakeholders in recognizing the value of PRO endpoints. In 2009, the FDA issued a guidance outlining how PROs could be used to support labeling claims. A year later, the EMA published a reflection paper on the same topic. Between 2006 and December 2010 44.8% of approved New Molecular Entities included PROs in pivotal studies (De Muro *et al.*, 2011). The inclusion of these endpoints in labeling occurred in only 24% of NMEs, demonstrating that the same rigor applied to primary endpoints is being applied to PROs in pivotal trials. While it is clear that clinical benefits demonstrated by PROs are recognized as valuable to a variety of stakeholders, the benefit of the inclusion of these data in product labeling versus other methods of dissemination (publication strategy) differs on a case by case basis. Developers must weigh the potential risks of over-complicating pivotal trials and potentially generating conflicting data by including PROs versus the potential benefits of PRO language appearing in the product label for enhanced market access and uptake.

Dose selection

Dose-response trials should be conducted in Phase II. Prior to initiating Phase III, there are a number of mechanisms to maximize the utility of previously generated data to inform and optimize Phase III dose selection. In the 2009 End of Phase IIa Meetings guidance, the FDA recommended the use of modeling and clinical trial simulations to analyze all prior data (from the early development program as well as from relevant external sources), quantify disease variability, and examine subgroup heterogeneity in order to select late-stage development doses. In addition, the use of PET imaging can characterize the relationship between dose, plasma concentration, and brain receptor occupancy (target) and can further support dose selection in CNS disorders. Dosing considerations in CNS are not significantly different than other therapeutic areas: dosing needs to optimize the benefit (efficacy)/risk (tolerability) profile for the majority of the population. Appropriate dose ranging performed in Phase II and the use of quantitative methodology should minimize the number of doses studied in Phase III. The number of doses required in Phase III, however, is likely compound-specific and dependent on the PK/PD profile of the molecule. A reasonable approach to Phase III therefore might include the minimum effective dose (MED) as well as a high dose defined by receptor occupancy or tolerability in the majority of the population.

Additional safety studies must also be conducted within Phase III to provide appropriate dosing instructions for special populations (e.g. renal or hepatic impaired, elderly, pediatrics). Regulators are committed to understanding the relationship between dosing/ exposure/tolerability and efficacy and have provided companies with several opportunities to discuss dose selection (End of Phase IIa, End of Phase II, and Type C meetings). No Phase III program should be conducted without prior agreement from health authorities that the quantitative methods utilized for dose selection were appropriate and that the Phase III dose range is sufficient to support approval.

Safety and tolerability

Despite the fact that the success rate in CNS drug development is alarmingly low, attrition due to unacceptable safety is less than 15% in this therapeutic area (Kola and Landis, 2004). This statistic supports the accuracy and efficiency of in vitro screening and animal models in predicting CNS toxicities early in the development process. Similar to dose selection, the management of safety evaluation in CNS is not significantly different from other therapeutic areas, and is not the major impediment to success in CNS development.

A primary goal of all drug development programs is to characterize the safety/ tolerability profile of a compound in relevant clinical populations and for durations consistent with its intended use. Attribution of adverse events to drug exposure defines a critical component of the risk-benefit assessment which drives the majority of development decisions including the ultimate fate of the compound as well as the dose. The Phase III database provides the majority of safety information used by most stakeholders to determine clinical utility. In general, databases contain 500–3000 subjects. In cases where benefit does not clearly outweigh risk, larger databases may be required. Placebo-controlled trials, which directly measure background adverse event rates, offer the most efficient means of assigning event causality to a drug and also serve to minimize exposure to non-tolerated compounds or doses. Alternatively, for diseases which affect only a small percentage of the overall population (e.g. orphan diseases) smaller safety databases may successfully support regulatory approval.

There is at least one emerging safety consideration that receives significant attention in CNS clinical trials: the prospective assessment of the occurrence of treatment-emergent suicidality. In the last 5 years, meta-analyses of antidepressant trials demonstrated that suicidality was a treatment-related adverse event in children (Hammad et al., 2006; Stone et al., 2009). In order to improve signal detection for such events in future development programs and meta-analyses, in 2010 the FDA issued a guidance requiring the prospective assessment of suicidality in all clinical trials involving any drugs being developed with CNS activity.

Conclusion

Phase III is the most costly component of the drug development process. Failure at this stage is a major disincentive to investment in drug development.

The multiple stakeholders involved and increased regulatory requirements have led more recently to larger, more complex, and more costly trials. This is particularly true for CNS programs.

The challenge for CNS drug developers is that to execute programs that address all these competing interests necessarily results in complexities that may be a barrier to recruitment, signal detection, and a successful outcome.

References

Akil, H., Brenner, S., Kandel, E., *et al.* (2010). The future of psychiatric research: genomes and neural circuits. *Science*, 327, 1580–81.

Arrowsmith, J. (2011). Trial watch: Phase III and submission failures: 2007–2010. *Nat Revs Drug Discov*, 10, 87.

Colagiuri, B. (2010). Participant expectancies in double blind randomized placebo controlled trials: potential limitations to trial validity. *Clinic Trials*, 1–10.

DeMuro, C., Clark, M., Mordin, M., *et al.* (2011). Reasons for rejection of PRO label claims: an analysis based on a review of PRO use among new molecular entities and biologic license applications 2006–2010. Poster at ISPOR 16th Annual International Meeting, May 21–25, Hilton Baltimore, Baltimore, MD, USA.

EMEA, C.F.M.P.F.H.U.C. reflection paper on the regulatory guidance for the use of health related quality of life (HRQL) measures in the evaluation of medicinal products. 16 March 2010.

FDA Guidance for Industry End-of-Phase IIa Meetings. US Department of Health and Human Services Food and Drug Administration Center for Drug Evaluation and Research (CDER), September 2009.

Guidance for Industry Suicidality: Prospective Assessment of Occurrence in Clinical Trials. US Department of Health and Human Services Food and Drug Administration Center for Drug Evaluation and Research (CDER), September 2010.

Hammad, T. A., Laughren, T., and Racoosin, J. (2006). Suicidality in pediatric patients treated with antidepressant drugs. *Arch Gen Psychiatr*, 63, 332–339.

International Conference on Harmonization (ICH) of Technical Requirements for Regulations of Pharmaceuticals for Human use. ICH Tripartite Guideline E-9 Document, Statistical Principles for Clinical trials, 5 February 1998.

Kemp, A. S., Schooler, N. R., Kalali, A. H., *et al.* (2010). What is causing the reduced drug–placebo difference in recent schizophrenia clinical trials and what can be done about it? *Schizophrenia Bull*, 36, 504–9.

Kinon, B. J., Potts, A. J., and Watson, S. B. (2011). Placebo response in clinical trials with schizophrenia patients. *Curr Opin Psychiat*, 24, 107–13.

Kola, I. and Landis, J. (2004). *Nat Rev Drug Discov*, 3, 711–15.

Paul, S. M., Mytelka, D. S., Dunwiddie, C. T., *et al.* (2010). How to improve R&D productivity: the pharmaceutical industry's grand challenge. *Nat Rev Drug Discov*, 9, 203–14.

Rush, A. J., Trivedi, M. H., Wisniewski, S. R. (2006a). Acute and longer-term outcomes in depressed outpatients requiring one or several treatment steps: a STAR*D Report. *Am J Psychiat*, 163, 1905–17.

Rush, A. J., Trivedi, M. H., Wisniewski, S. R., *et al.* (2006b). STAR*D Study Team. Bupropion-SR, sertraline, or venlafaxine-XR after failure of SSRIs for depression. *New Engl J Med*, 354, 1231–42.

Stone, M., Laughren, T., Jones, M. L., *et al.* (2009). Risk of suicidality in clinical trials of antidepressants in adults: analysis of proprietary data submitted to US Food and Drug Administration, *Brit Med J*, 339, 2880.

Targum, S., Pollack, M., and Fava, M. (2008). Redefining affective disorders: relevance for drug development. *CNS Neurosci Therapeut*, 14, 2–9.

Walsh, B. T., Seidman, S. N., Sysko, R., and Gould, M. (2002). Placebo response in studies of major depression: variable, substantial, and growing. *J Am Med Assoc*, 287, 1840–47.

Wisniewski, S. R., Rush, A. J., Nierenberg, A. A., *et al.* (2009). Can Phase III trial results of antidepressant medications be generalized to clinical practice? A STAR*D Report. *Am J Psychiat*, 166, 599–607.

Statistics issues relevant to CNS drug development

Craig H. Mallinckrodt, William R. Prucka, and
Geert Molenberghs

Introduction

In diseases of the central nervous system (CNS) only 9% of the drugs that enter Phase I testing receive regulatory approval, which is lower than all other therapeutic areas except oncology. Approximately 50% of compound attrition is due to not demonstrating efficacy in Phase II, which is a 15% increase compared with the previous decade (Hurko and Ryan, 2005). Meanwhile, the attrition rate of CNS drugs in Phase III is about 50% (Kola and Landis, 2004). And even for drugs that are approved many trials fail to show efficacy. Together, these findings point to high rates of false-negative and false-positive efficacy results as a major obstacle in CNS drug development.

Statistical issues such as the experimental design and the method of analysis are inherent to discussions regarding false-negative and false-positive results. Many manuscripts and text books have been written on the design and analysis of clinical trials. See for example Piantadosi (2005). Much is known about optimizing designs for individual clinical trials. However, drug development involves a series of studies, and optimizing each individual trial in a series does not necessarily optimize the series of studies. And optimizing each individual compound in a portfolio does not necessarily optimize the portfolio.

Therefore, the focus of this chapter is on optimizing the series of studies, efficacy studies in particular, required to develop a drug. Consideration is given to design archetypes – a general framework to categorize development approaches, along with the use of positive controls, early comparisons between a test drug and a standard of care (SoC), and to modeling and simulation of entire portfolios of drugs. Issues of particular importance to individual trials in CNS, such as placebo response and missing data, are also covered.

Design archetypes

Phase II studies play an important role in optimizing clinical drug development because this is the phase when efficacy is typically first evaluated. The correctness of Phase II results dictates the effectiveness and efficiency of development programs. False-negative results mistakenly terminate the development of effective therapies. False-positive results mistakenly trigger large, expensive, but futile Phase III programs. Optimizing the design of Phase II studies must be done in conjunction with optimizing Phase III/IV studies, and the Phase II plan implies certain goals must be reached in Phase I to support the subsequent studies. In addition, given that Phase II is the middle of the three phases

Essential CNS Drug Development, ed. A. Kalali, Sheldon Preskorn, J. Kwentus, and Stephen M. Stahl.
Published by Cambridge University Press. © Cambridge University Press 2012.

required for marketing approval, it is a focal point for achieving objectives sequentially, in parallel, or seamlessly via adaptive approaches.

Phase II studies explore efficacy for the targeted indication (i.e., establish proof of concept (PoC)) and assess the dose-response relationship (ICH Guidelines: E4). One way to approach Phase II is to establish PoC and assess dose-response in separate, sequential studies. For test drugs that are not effective, sequential studies can be more efficient because resources are not wasted studying multiple doses of a test drug, none of which are useful. For test drugs that are effective, the sequential approach may be slow and inefficient. For example, it could take many years to plan and conduct sequential PoC and dose-finding studies, and the treatment arms from the PoC study will likely again be tested in the dose-finding study. Thus, the sequential study approach leads to efficient terminations, but inefficient approvals (Mallinckrodt *et al.*, 2010a).

Another way to approach Phase II is to conduct a single study focusing on dose finding that is also used to establish PoC. As previously noted, for test drugs that are not effective, this approach is inefficient. But if the drug is effective, more information is obtained sooner and at lower cost than by going through the sequence of PoC followed by dose finding. Therefore, this approach leads to efficient approvals, but inefficient terminations (Mallinckrodt *et al.*, 2010a).

The optimum Phase II design for a particular drug therefore hinges on whether or not that drug is effective, a characteristic of course unknown when Phase II studies are designed because establishing efficacy is one of the objectives. Hence, understanding and mitigating the trade-off between efficient termination/inefficient approval (quick kill) and inefficient termination/efficient approval (quick win) approaches is a key to drug development.

Axes of development

An over-arching framework for optimizing the design of Phase II studies in CNS disorders has been proposed for scenarios where dose response is relevant to clinical practice (Mallinckrodt *et al.*, 2010a). The authors explained their approach as follows:

> It is assumed dose response is relevant when opportunity exists to fine-tune dosing on an individual patient basis. For example, in acute symptomatic treatments of chronic diseases, such as pain, migraine, depression, anxiety, attention-deficit hyperactivity disorder, and schizophrenia dosing can start low and go slow. In areas where response to treatment is slow, or where the treatment goal is to prevent worsening, such as disease modification treatments for Alzheimer's disease (AD), little flexibility may exist to adjust dosing based on efficacy. In these situations that require long evaluation periods, by the time a patient is identified as not responding adequately to the initial dose it may be too late to consider alternatives.

> In scenarios where dose response is relevant in clinical practice development can be optimized by considering two factors – termed the axes of development: (1) the optimism for success; and, (2) signal detection. Optimism is essentially the probability that the test drug is effective, or p(E). Signal detection refers to assay sensitivity – the ability of a study to detect a difference between treatments when a difference truly exists. A third axis, external factors (such as logistic or financial considerations) is also important, but idiosyncratic to each compound and therefore not part of the over-arching principles that influence all compounds.

> Although optimism for efficacy can be measured on a continuum as p(E), for simplicity the authors categorized optimism as high or low. Optimism was considered high if the mechanism of

Table 1. Axes of development and their drug development implications

		Signal unlikely to exist	Signal likely to exist
	High ($\Delta >= 0.5$)	Easy to find signal if it exists	Easy to find signal if it exists
		Showing dose response possible	Showing dose response possible
Signal detection			
	Low ($\Delta < 0.5$)	Signal unlikely to exist	Signal likely to exist
		Not easy to find signal if it exists	Not easy to find signal if it exists
		Showing dose response difficult	Showing dose response difficult
		Low	**High**
		Optimism	

Table reused with permission from *Drug Information Journal.*

action of the test drug had been established as effective or if a biomarker result indicative of efficacy had been obtained in Phase I. Optimism was considered low if the mechanism of action was novel.

Signal detection is strongly influenced by the magnitude of the treatment effect. Therefore, signal detection can also be measured on a continuum, based on effect size. However, again for simplicity, a cut off for high versus low signal detection was chosen, based on an effect size of 0.5 standard deviations.

The 2 × 2 cross tabulation of optimism and signal detection categorized as high or low are summarized in Table 1 with their drug development implications. An important point in the table is that when the signal is small, assessing dose response is likely to be more difficult. To illustrate, consider scenario A where the maximally effective dose yields an effect size of 0.60; in scenario B, the corresponding effect size is 0.30. In scenario A the dose yielding 50% of the maximal effect has an effect size of 0.3 and the difference between that dose and the maximally effective dose is also an effect size of 0.3. In scenario A, the difference between doses is as great as the difference between the maximally effective dose and placebo in scenario B. In scenario B, larger sample sizes are required to achieve a commensurate level of reliability on the same evaluation. A dose-ranging study in scenario B would require a large sample size, which might be a poor investment if it were as yet not proven that any of the doses had a beneficial effect.

Primary archetypes

Mallinckrodt *et al.* (2010a) used the implications outlined in Table 1 to suggest two primary design archetypes.

(1) *Fast-to-PoC*. This archetype focuses on fast, efficient termination. If optimism is low, the drug is more likely to be ineffective than to be effective. Hence, it makes sense to focus on a design that quickly and cheaply tests whether or not the drug has any

beneficial effect. It also makes sense to not try and show a dose-response early in development if it is more likely that no doses are effective and/or if showing dose-response in effective drugs is unlikely owing to small effect sizes.

(2) *Fast-to-registration.* This archetype focuses on fast, efficient approval. If success is more likely, the overall clinical plan may be accelerated to rapidly achieve the ultimate goal of regulatory approval. In Phase II, it makes sense to focus on a design that quickly characterizes dose response, if the anticipated effect size is sufficient such that showing dose response is possible, because many subsequent studies require knowledge of dose response.

These primary archetypes were mapped to the axes of development. The fast-to-registration archetype fits well for scenarios where signal detection and optimism are both high – the upper right quadrant of Table 1. Fast-to-PoC fits well for scenarios where signal detection and optimism are both low – the lower left quadrant of Table 1. However, further elaboration is needed to understand how to best map primary archetypes to those scenarios where one of the axes is low and the other is high.

Secondary archetypes

Determining the proper archetype for scenarios where one axis is high and the other is low is accomplished via selection of an appropriate secondary archetype (Mallinckrodt *et al.*, 2010a). The secondary archetype will often be a hybrid of the two primary archetypes; consequently, this is a fertile area for adaptive designs. For simplicity in describing the following secondary archetypes, define a PoC study as two-arm, focusing on a high dose, a forced titration to the maximally tolerated dose, or a flexible dose of the test drug versus placebo; define a dose-ranging study as including placebo and at least three fixed doses of the test drug. Secondary archetypes for a fast-to-PoC approach may include:

1. *Separate PoC and dose-finding studies in Phase II.* This scenario is slow because it employs two sequential trials and is inefficient because treatment arms from the PoC study (high dose and placebo) are repeated in the dose-ranging study. However, this approach discharges risk at low cost because a decision for further development is based on the first, small trial.

2. *PoC in Phase II, with a dose-finding study in Phase III.* Secondary archetypes 1 and 2 involve the same studies. However, the availability of pivotal clinical-trial material or some bridging strategy results in the dose-ranging study in secondary archetype 2 counting as one of the pivotal studies in Phase III required for regulatory approval.

3. *PoC in Phase II, with multiple studies using overlapping doses in Phase III to assess dose response.* This approach can be especially useful when effect sizes are small and therefore the number per arm needed to assess dose response is large.

4. *Seamless adaptive Phase IIa/IIb study, focusing first on PoC and then after a positive signal is found at an interim analysis, patient allocation is altered to focus on dose finding.*

Secondary archetypes for a fast-to-registration approach include:

1. *Single dose-finding study in Phase II.* This approach is useful in the high signal detection scenarios when effect sizes are larger as the larger effect sizes mean that sample size per

arm for a given power is small. The 2- to 3-fold increase in total sample size typically needed for a dose-ranging study versus a PoC trial may be, for example, the difference between total enrollment of 200 patients and 80 patients, respectively. The additional 120 patients may be justifiable to obtain dose response from the same study that establishes PoC, especially if it is likely that the drug is effective.

2. *Skip Phase II altogether.* This strategy might be employed when confidence for efficacy is very high, such as when a well-validated biomarker or healthy volunteer model is used in Phase I to establish PoC (and perhaps also dose response). While such a scenario may be difficult to achieve, the advantages are compelling.

3. *Seamless adaptive Phase IIa/IIb study, focusing first on PoC and then after a positive signal is found at an interim analysis patient allocation is altered to focus on dose finding.* This is essentially the same scenario as examined for secondary archetype 4 in the fast to PoC primary archetype.

4. *Seamless adaptive Phase II/III study focusing first on dose response then dropping arms and proceeding to Phase III.* This is similar to secondary archetype 1 except that rather than doing separate dose-finding and confirmatory studies the dose-finding portion seamlessly transitions into the confirmatory phase (Mallinckrodt *et al.*, 2010b).

Context

The archetypes noted above focus on a limited set of scenarios: acute-phase clinical trials where dose response is relevant in treating individual patients. The axes of development, defined by optimism for success and signal detection, provide the over-arching framework from which primary and secondary archetypes are defined to guide individual design decisions.

The key distinction between primary archetypes is whether the first efficacy study should focus on establishing PoC (fast-to-PoC) or on evaluating dose response (fast-to-registration). Secondary archetypes are used to minimize the trade-offs between the efficient-kill-inefficient-win fast-to-PoC archetype and the inefficient-kill-efficient-win fast-to-registration archetype.

These archetypes are not an all-encompassing list, nor do they provide specific recommendations for specific scenarios. Rather, the focus is on the key concepts that provide the over-arching framework from which decisions can be made.

Portfolio perspective

Improving the quality of studies that first establish efficacy has been cited as the most important factor in reducing the attrition rate in drug development (Kola and Landis, 2004). Although the design of PoC studies is complex and difficult in its own right, PoC studies cannot be designed in isolation without considering other studies. The central premise to optimizing drug development is that optimizing each in a series of studies does not optimize the series.

Hence, that which is optimum for an individual drug may not be optimum for the portfolio. For example, assume a large dose-response study is twice as costly as a smaller two-arm PoC study. While a dose-response study might be optimum for drug X, it may not be optimum for the portfolio if the extra resources devoted to drug X takes away the opportunity to study another drug.

Adaptive designs

Adaptive design of clinical trials is a rapidly evolving area. Extensive examination of adaptive designs and their relevance to drug development is available (Chow and Chang, 2007). As noted in several of the secondary design archetypes, adaptive designs may play an important role in drug development. For example, an adaptive design may mitigate the trade-offs between the fast-to-PoC and fast-to-registration approach by initially randomizing mostly to the maximum dose and placebo, thereby achieving an efficient determination of PoC; and after a positive interim result, allocation can be altered and/or dose arms added to explore dose response, thereby providing in an expeditious manner the dose-response information needed for subsequent development. This approach is explored in more detail in the following example.

Consider a test drug with three dose levels (low, mid, high) to be evaluated against placebo. The intent of this drug's Phase II development is to determine if any of the three doses are effective, and, if so, determine which dose(s) to carry forward into Phase III. For illustration, two secondary archetypes within the fast-to-PoC primary archetype were compared.

The first approach used secondary archetype 1, the two-trial "sequential" approach where initially a small PoC trial compared high dose versus placebo. Conditional on success in this trial, a larger dose-ranging trial was conducted. For simplicity it was assumed that if the initial PoC trial was successful, failure in the dose-ranging trial did not halt development. This approach is expected to provide an efficient kill for ineffective drugs, but can be inefficient for drugs that are effective.

The second approach used secondary archetype 4, a single two-stage "seamless" PoC/dose-ranging adaptive design. The intent of the adaption was to mitigate the efficiency trade-offs from the sequential approach so that the study could be reasonably efficient regardless of whether or not the drug was effective. In the seamless approach stage 1 focused on establishing evidence of efficacy (PoC) by primarily randomizing to the highest dose and placebo. If the drug was sufficiently promising (i.e. not futile), stage 2 was initiated wherein randomization probabilities were altered to focus more on lower and mid doses, thereby exploring dose response.

The sequential and seamless approaches as implemented here also differed in the level of proof required to continue development. The sequential approach included traditional powering and type I error requiring fairly conclusive evidence the drug was effective in order to continue development. For the seamless approach development continued to stage 2 so long as futility had not been clearly established in stage 1.

For analysis, baseline and endpoint (continuous) outcomes were simulated to mimic outcomes in acute pain disorders where lower scores indicate lower symptom severity. Contrasts were constructed such that negative change scores indicated improvement. The standard deviation in changes from baseline was 2.0. A clinically meaningful difference (CMD) was defined as a mean difference of -0.5 for test drug versus placebo.

Two dose-response scenarios were evaluated. In the first, no doses were effective as each dose and placebo had a mean -1.0 point change to endpoint. In the second scenario (high dose effective) the mean endpoint changes were -1.0, -1.25, -1.4, and -2.0 for placebo, low, mid, and high doses, respectively. Therefore, only the high dose had a CMD versus placebo, with an effect size of 0.5. A Bayesian analysis was used to evaluate the likelihood of both success and futility. Success was defined as at least one dose having a 60% or greater probability of achieving or exceeding the CMD. Futility was defined as all doses having less than a 25% probability of attaining the CMD. In practice, these values must be carefully chosen taking into consideration resource constraints, the expected value of the drug, the cost of Phase III failure, and other factors. Too lax a futility criterion will result in frequent false-positive findings wherein ineffective drugs are passed into large, subsequent studies that are destined for failure. Too high a futility hurdle will result in many false-negative findings wherein effective drugs are mistakenly terminated.

For all scenarios 1000 trials were simulated using the Fixed and Adaptive Clinical Trial Simulator (FACTS) software. In the sequential approach the initial PoC trial had 70 patients per arm; comparable to a non-Bayesian trial with 90% power and an alpha level of 5% against placebo in pairwise comparisons (that does not incorporate the CMD). If successful, the PoC trial was followed by a dose-ranging trial with 210 subjects with fixed allocation and without interim analyses. For the seamless approach, an interim analysis was conducted at the end of stage 1 and after each block of 10 patients. Results were compared against futility criteria and to adaptively alter the allocation. The adaptive allocation strategy placed increased probability for patients to be assigned to the most effective doses, therefore providing more information on doses likely to achieve the CMD. Placebo was not adaptively allocated, and was set at a fixed 1/3 probability throughout the second stage of the study. Three different allocation strategies for stage 1 were tested, each allocating a different proportion of subjects to the high-dose group (described in Table 2). The average sample size for the scenarios when the drug was and was not effective was determined for each approach along with the probability of success for the high-dose effective scenario and the rate of false-positive results for the no-dose effective scenario.

The results in Table 2 indicate that for scenarios where the drug was effective, the sequential approach yielded an average sample size of 323.1 patients, with a success rate of 87.2%. In the seamless approach the corresponding average sample size was 205. Of the various seamless approaches tested, the maximum unequal allocation approach performed the best, with an 89.3% success rate. When no doses were effective, the sequential approach averaged 149.9 patients, and falsely declared success in 4.5% of the trials. The best seamless approach averaged 139.6 patients with a false-positive rate of 6.1%.

Therefore, in this example, the seamless approach with maximum unequal allocation and a low hurdle for continuing into stage 2 terminated ineffective drugs approximately as efficiently as the sequential approach and correctly declared drugs effective and provided dose-response information with less than 2/3 the patients used in the sequential approach (323 vs. 205).

This example illustrates the benefits of quantitative evaluation of design alternatives. It is not a specific recommendation. Many potential dose-response scenarios and futility rules could be considered and the seamless approach is not necessarily optimal. Also, the optimal allocation for stage 1 is likely situation-dependent. It may not always be optimal to randomize primarily to the highest dose, particularly when tolerability is considered.

Moreover, an adaptive design likely involves added expense. Non-trivial operational expenses associated with adaptive allocation, study drug supply, and futility monitoring must be considered. For additional considerations regarding adaptive designs in clinical trials see Gallo et al. (2006).

Use of positive controls

Active comparators may be included in addition to a test drug and placebo in clinical trials as positive controls to assess assay sensitivity; that is, to determine whether the study

Table 2. Average sample size and success rate of a two-stage adaptive design for proof of concept and dose ranging when the high dose is effective and when no doses are effective

| Dose response | Design | Average sample size | | | | | | % Success |
		Total	Placebo	Low dose	Mid dose	High dose	
High dose effective	Equal allocation*	204.4	83.1	28.0	31.7	61.6	84.50%
	Mid unequal allocation**	205.9	83.6	21.2	26.2	74.9	87.10%
	Max unequal allocation***	205.0	83.3	19.8	20.1	81.8	89.30%
	PoC + dose ranging****	323.1	131.0	40.1	41.0	111.0	87.20%
No dose effective	Equal allocation	157.0	67.3	30.8	29.8	29.0	7.90%
	Mid unequal allocation	161.7	69.0	25.0	26.1	41.7	8.40%
	Max unequal allocation	139.6	61.5	13.4	11.6	53.1	6.10%
	PoC + dose ranging	149.5	73.2	2.1	2.1	72.1	4.50%

* Stage 1 allocation of (45, 15, 15, 15) for (Placebo, Low, Mid, High) followed by adaptive allocation, maximum $n = 210$.
** Stage 1 allocation of (45, 5, 10, 45) followed by adaptive allocation, maximum $n = 210$.
*** Stage 1 allocation of (45, 0, 0, 45) followed by adaptive allocation, maximum $n = 210$.
**** PoC trial allocated (70, 0, 0, 70), if successful, fixed dose ranging trial with $n = 210$ allocated (70, 46, 47, 47).

provided a valid test of the experimental drug. Therefore, including positive controls has intuitive appeal as a means to foster better decisions from a trial. However, intuitive appeal is not a substitute for quantitative evaluation when assessing if, and if so when, it is useful to include positive controls to assess assay sensitivity in CNS trials.

Quantitative evaluation

Mallinckrodt *et al.* (2010b) used a numerical analysis of hypothetical examples to assess the utility of positive controls. The key findings of that study suggested that positive controls are not always beneficial. These authors concluded that across a series of studies, if positive controls are to be useful more often than not, they must have at least 80% power and preferably 90% power for their contrast with placebo; and, positive controls are more likely to be useful as the likelihood the test drug is effective decreases. The authors illustrated these conclusions via the following examples and tables.

Assume an effective test drug and a positive control are compared with placebo and correctly powered at 80%. Since both drugs are effective, the correct result would be for both drugs to yield a significant difference from placebo. But with 80% power each drug is expected to be

Table 3. Probabilities of outcomes when the test drug is effective and the positive control and the test drug are powered at 80% – assuming independence of outcomes

		Significance of positive control		Total
		Yes	No	
Significance of test drug				
	Yes	64	16	80
	No	16	4	20
Total		80	20	

Cell values are the percentage of trials expected to yield the various outcomes under the assumed conditions.
Table reused with permission from *Drug Information Journal.*

non-significant simply due to chance alone in 20% of the trials. If the tests are independent, then the probabilities of two joint outcomes are the product of the individual probabilities. The probabilities of all possible outcomes from this hypothetical scenario are summarized in Table 3.

In this scenario, 64% (.80 *.80) of the trials are expected to yield a significant difference for both the test drug and the positive control. Therefore, at least one "wrong" result is expected in 36% (100%−64%) of the trials. More specifically, in 16% (.8 *.2) of the trials only the test drug is expected to be significant. In another 16% (.2 *.8) only the positive control is expected to be significant, and in 4% (.2 *.2) neither is expected to be significant.

Now assume each drug is powered at 50% rather than 80%. The correct result would again be for both drugs to yield a significant difference from placebo. However, only 25% (.5 *.5 = .25) of the trials are expected to yield a significant difference for both drugs. Therefore, at least one "wrong" result is expected in 75% of the trials.

In scenarios where the test drug is not effective (test drug equal to placebo), the correct result would be for the positive control to yield a significant difference and for the test drug to be not significant. However, due to chance alone, the test drug is expected to be significant in 5% of the trials (with one-tailed alpha = .05 the false positive rate is 5%) and the positive control is expected to be not significant in 20% of the trials if powered at 80%.

Hence, assuming independence of outcomes, 4% (.05 *.8) of the trials are expected to yield a significant difference for both drugs, and the test drug only is expected to be significant in 1% of trials. The correct result (test drug not significant and positive control significant) is expected in 76% of trials. Therefore, at least one "wrong" result is expected in 24% of the trials.

If power for the positive control is lowered to 50%, as might be the case when randomizing fewer patients to the positive control than to the test drug, or in disease states where known active compounds frequently fail, even with large sample sizes, the correct result of the test drug being non-significant with the positive control significant is expected in only 47.5% of the trials. Therefore, at least one "wrong" result is expected in 52.5% of the trials (Mallinckrodt *et al.*, 2010b).

Mallinckrodt *et al.* (2010b) further illustrated the implications of correct and incorrect findings from positive control arms of Phase II studies on drug development. They assumed that if the test drug was significant then development proceeded to Phase III; if the test drug was not significant and the positive control was significant, then development was stopped; if neither the test drug nor the positive control was significant, then the PoC trial was repeated.

Positive control outcomes were classified as neutral, helpful, or harmful. Consider first those scenarios when the test drug is in fact effective. Positive controls were said to have a neutral effect whenever the test drug separates from placebo because the correct answer was obtained for the test drug and the positive control does not add information. When the effective test drug fails to separate, the positive control was said to be harmful when it separates from placebo because it reinforces the false-negative result by suggesting the study was capable of finding a difference from placebo for the test drug if a difference existed. The positive control was said to be helpful when it does not separate from placebo because it suggests that the study did not adequately evaluate the test drug.

Mallinckrodt *et al.* (2010b) used the results in Table 4 to summarize probabilities of various outcomes and their drug development implications, along with utility of the positive control for those scenarios where the test drug is effective. The probabilities in Table 4 are different from the probabilities in Table 3 because they accounted for the correlation in outcomes from comparing the test drug and positive control to the same placebo group whereas the probabilities in Table 3 assumed independence of outcomes in order to make the initial illustration of concepts simpler.

The probabilities that the positive control had a helpful, neutral, or harmful effect were 0.087, 0.800, and 0.113, respectively. Thus, in these scenarios where the test drug was effective, the positive control was seldom beneficial, just as often harmful, but always increased the cost of the studies.

Similar calculations were performed for scenarios where the test drug was not effective and are summarized in Table 5. When the test drug and positive control separated from placebo, the positive control reinforced the false-positive result. When the test drug did not separate from placebo and the positive control did, the positive control helped because it provided more confidence that the study was capable of finding an effect of the test drug if an effect existed. When neither drug separated from placebo, the positive control was harmful because it erroneously suggested that the study was not capable of finding a difference when in fact the study failed simply due to random change, the lack of 100% power. The probabilities that the positive control had a helpful or harmful effect were 0.751 and 0.249, respectively, with the positive control never having a neutral effect, but again always adding to the cost of the studies (Mallinckrodt *et al.*, 2010b).

Portfolio perspective

Mallinckrodt *et al.* (2010b) also considered the impact of positive controls over an entire portfolio of drugs and those results are summarized in Table 6.

> When the positive control was powered at 80%, with 50% of the test drugs being effective, the frequencies of the positive control having a beneficial, neutral, or harmful effect across the portfolio were 42%, 40%, and 18%, respectively. When powered at 80% with 33.3% of the test drugs being effective the corresponding percentages were 53%, 27%, and 20%.

> When the positive control was powered at 90%, with 50% of the test drugs being effective, the frequencies of a positive control having a beneficial, neutral, or harmful effect were 45%, 40%, and 15%, respectively. When powered at 90% with 33.3% of the test drugs being effective the corresponding percentages were 58%, 27%, and 15%.

> And thus, while use of positive controls has intuitive appeal for fostering better inferences, careful consideration reveals the following conundrum. Positive controls are thought to be useful when assay sensitivity is low because it is difficult to trust the results of the study, especially negative

Table 4. Probabilities of outcomes and their consequences when the test drug is effective and the positive control and the test drug are powered at 80% – not assuming independence

Active outcome	Test outcome	Result/ decision	Probability[1]	Action	Utility of active arm	Cost/gain
Y	Y	True positive	0.687	Proceed to Phase III	Neutral	Unneeded arm in PoC study
Y	N	False negative	0.113	Kill drug	Harmful	Opportunity for new treatment lost
N	Y	True positive	0.113	Proceed to Phase III	Neutral	Unneeded arm in PoC study
N	N	No decision	0.087	Repeat PoC	Helpful	Opportunity for new treatment preserved

[1] Cell values are the probabilities that a trial is expected to yield the various outcomes under the assumed conditions. Table reused with permission from *Drug Information Journal*.

Table 5. Probabilities of outcomes and their consequences when the test drug is not effective and the positive control is powered at 80% – not assuming independence

Active outcome	Test outcome	Result/ decision	Probability[1]	Action	Utility of active arm	Cost
Y	Y	False positive	0.049	Proceed to Phase III	Harmful	Expensive, futile Phase III
Y	N	True negative	0.751	Kill drug	Helpful	None
N	Y	False positive	0.001	Proceed to Phase III	Harmful	Expensive, futile Phase III
N	N	No decision	0.199	Repeat PoC	Harmful	Repeat futile PoC

[1] Cell values are the probabilities that a trial is expected to yield the various outcomes under the assumed conditions. Table reused with permission from *Drug Information Journal*.

results for a test drug. But including a positive control may not improve decision-making since the results from the positive control are also unreliable. On the other hand, if assay sensitivity is good, results of the study can be trusted, including results from the test drug, thereby negating the need for a positive control (Mallinckrodt *et al.*, 2010b).

General conclusions from simplistic examples are an instructive starting point. Namely, positive controls are more likely to be useful as the probability the test drug is effective decreases and as the power for the positive control increases. Therefore, positive control arms should be powered at a minimum of 80%, and preferably 90%.

Table 6. Frequencies of neutral, helpful, and harmful outcomes of positive controls

	Positive control powered at			
	80%		90%	
	Percentage of test drugs effective		Percentage of test drugs effective	
	50%	33.3%	50%	33.3%
Positive control helped	42%	53%	45%	58%
Positive control neutral	40%	27%	40%	27%
Positive control hurt	18%	20%	15%	15%

Assume an infinitely large number of compounds are tested, and the percentage of compounds that are effective is either 50% or 33.3%.
Table reused with permission from *Drug Information Journal*.

However, this simplistic viewpoint ignores the opportunity cost associated with including a positive control. Direct costs of including a positive control are not trivial: the drug must be blinded, stability-tested, packaged, distributed, and tested in patients. But the results from the positive control only indirectly inform us about the test drug. The resources devoted to a positive control could alternatively be used to study another test drug. Moreover, positive controls assess assay sensitivity, they do not improve it. Two studies of test drug and placebo instead of one study that also includes a positive control may improve assay sensitivity with little to no increase in the total sample size or cost (Mallinckrodt *et al.*, 2010b).

The key question to address is if the benefit from including a positive control for study of drug X is greater than the benefit that could be had if those resources were devoted to studying another drug or to another study of drug X.

Early comparisons with standard of care

One of the changes in recent years in the healthcare industry is that key stakeholders are demanding evidence not only that new drugs are safe and effective, but that they are safer or more effective than alternatives. Perhaps this is a natural consequence of an ever-increasing availability of generic drugs. Therefore, greater need exists to understand the risks and benefits of a test drug compared with a standard of care (SoC). Ideally, this information would be available early in development because even if a test drug were superior to placebo in a PoC study, it may not be worthwhile to continue developing the drug unless it also provides benefit beyond a cheaper, generic therapy (Mallinckrodt *et al.*, 2010c).

However, efficacy comparisons versus SoC in a PoC study can be challenging (Lieberman *et al.*, 2005; Temple and Ellenberg, 2000). For example, reliably establishing a difference between a test drug and SoC typically requires an appreciably larger sample size to achieve a given level of power than when comparing the test drug with placebo because the SoC is superior to placebo.

The larger sample size required to compare a test drug with SoC has important implications for drug development. Given that many drugs tested in PoC studies will have no benefit, that is, they are not better than placebo, it may not be ethical or financially feasible to do a big trial to compare the test drug with SoC when a small study would show the test drug was not different from placebo. Alternatively, a smaller study to compare with placebo may not be meaningful when SoC is the benchmark that really matters.

In comparing a test drug and SoC we may assume that having some data is better than having no data; including even a few patients in an active comparator arm in a PoC trial is useful for benchmarking the test drug versus the SoC. However, including an active comparator adds cost and potentially logistic or methodological difficulties to the study. Hence, it is important to explicitly evaluate the utility of the comparisons vs. SoC (Mallinckrodt *et al.*, 2010c).

Quantitative evaluation

Mallinckrodt *et al.* (2010c) used an analytic study to determine the reliability of various sample sizes and criteria for comparing a test drug with SoC in scenarios patterned after CNS clinical trials. Several criteria for superiority were considered because definitive hypothesis tests for superiority of the test drug versus SoC likely lead to prohibitively large sample sizes, especially for a PoC study. Thus, in addition to the probability of a significant result on a superiority test, the probabilities of establishing non-inferiority of the test drug were also considered along with the probability of properly ranking the test drug and SoC.

As expected, superiority testing maintained the desired rate of false-positive results, but yielded high rates of false-negative results even when sample sizes were 5-fold greater than what was needed to have adequate power for comparisons versus placebo. Non-inferiority testing and rankings yielded high rates of false-positive results (continuing development when the test drug was not superior to SoC) at all sample sizes. It was still possible to establish non-inferiority since the two treatments were in fact equal. With a sample size 5-fold greater than needed for adequate power versus placebo, the probability of establishing non-inferiority was approximately 50%.

This demonstrates a difficulty in using non-inferiority as the basis for continuing development when superiority is the goal. Namely, if the test drug is not really better than SoC, non-inferiority tests when used as a less stringent assessment of potential for superiority can lead to many false conclusions that the test drug has potential to be superior. Moreover, the larger the sample size, the more likely is this type of false-positive result.

Using rankings also led to many false-positive results when the true difference between test drug and SoC was zero. The probability of getting a point estimate of exactly zero difference between the experimental drug and SoC is negligible, and each drug will be ranked as better than the other half the time, leading to a false-positive rate of 50% regardless of sample size.

It is also important to consider that constructing valid comparisons versus SoC may require extensive experience with the test drug (Leiberman *et al.*, 2005). When first assessing efficacy, (1) the dose of the test drug may not be the most appropriate dose to compare with SoC; (2) the most relevant patient population may not have been enrolled; or (3) the most relevant outcomes on which to focus may not be known. Therefore, the value of comparing a test drug versus SoC in a PoC study is difficult to ascertain (Mallinckrodt *et al.*, 2010c).

Only a few of the many scenarios and criteria for comparing a test drug with SoC were considered by Mallinckrodt *et al.* (2010c). Therefore, the main point from that work is not the specific outcomes, such as 5-fold more patients required to get a reliable comparison vs. SoC than for a contrast with placebo. Rather, the focus is on the general point that comparisons versus SoC take much larger studies than comparisons with placebo.

Portfolio perspective

To contemplate the consequences of early comparisons versus SoC for a portfolio of drugs, Mallinckrodt *et al.* (2010c) considered a hypothetical scenario similar to the one below where research and development costs are thought of as the opportunity to buy outcomes, with only a fixed amount that can be spent.

Obviously, various strategies might be leveraged to buy outcomes more efficiently, but ultimately only so many outcomes can be bought. Further, assume that some outcomes are more expensive than others. For example, assume contrasts versus SoC are 3-fold more costly than contrasts versus placebo since the sample sizes required are larger. In other words, assume comparisons with placebo cost 1 unit and comparisons with SoC cost 3 units. Also assume that the research budget allows purchase of 20 outcome units.

If all PoC studies contain SoC, it would cost 4 units to evaluate each compound (1 unit for the placebo outcome and 3 units for the SoC outcome). Hence, 5 compounds could be evaluated in total. If no PoC studies contained SoC, 10 compounds could be initially screened versus placebo, costing 10 units, for example. Then, assuming three compounds were positive they would then be evaluated versus SoC, costing an additional 9 units. In this hypothetical situation, would it be better to rigorously compare five compounds versus placebo and SoC, or would it be better to preliminarily evaluate 10 drugs versus placebo and only proceed to comparing versus SoC for those compounds that beat placebo, or is some combination of the approaches optimal?

The optimal solution is probably influenced by the probability that the test drug is effective. For test drugs with proven mechanisms of action it is more likely that the compounds have some benefit and thus first testing versus placebo would not screen out many compounds. And there is likely greater need to compare versus SoC as early as possible since already proven compounds of the same mechanism are available. Conversely, for test drugs with novel mechanisms, it is less likely that they will have any beneficial effect and a small trial versus placebo will screen out many compounds. Moreover, if the novel test drug happens to beat placebo, it is likely to differ in some meaningful way from the SoC because it has a different mechanism.

The key point is that comparisons versus SoC are costly and in a resource-constrained environment will result in the ability to evaluate fewer drugs. On the other hand, spending all the time and money required to fully develop a test drug only to find out it has no meaningful benefit over a cheap generic drug is perhaps the most wasteful scenario of all.

Historical data

In scenarios where adequately powered concurrent controls are not efficient, historical data may be useful. Use of historical control as opposed to, or in addition to, concurrent control is essentially a trade-off between bias and precision. If the bias in the historical control can be minimized and sufficient historical data exist so that the effects can be estimated precisely, historical control can be useful (Mallinckrodt *et al.*, 2010c).

Bayesian statistical approaches can explicitly utilize historical data for indirect comparisons or incorporate historical data and concurrent data into the analysis (Berry and Stangl, 1996; Spiegelhalter *et al.*, 2004). In a Bayesian analysis with concurrent control, prior information (the historical data) is combined with the current data to estimate the drug effect. This estimate is termed the posterior estimate and it is often expressed as a probability of the true effect falling within a certain interval; for example, a 95% probability that the true treatment effect is between X and Y.

The posterior estimate is a weighted average of the prior and current data, with weightings determined by the amount of information in historical data relative to the current data. When the amount of historical data contributing to the prior estimate is large, especially as compared to the sample size of the current data, the prior is said to be informative and it contributes more to the posterior estimate than if prior data are less abundant. As sample size of the current data increases relative to the prior data, the posterior estimate is more heavily influenced by the current data and the prior data may have a negligible effect.

When the prior and current data reflect a similar magnitude of treatment effect, Bayesian methods have increased power over traditional techniques, essentially augmenting the sample size of the current data with additional (historical) data. For example, consider a study comparing a test drug to placebo with an effect size of 0.5. For 90% power on a one-sided superiority test with a type I error rate of 5%, 70 subjects per arm would be needed. Under these same circumstances including prior data that indicates a 95% probability that the true effect size is between 0 and 1, 56 subjects per arm would be needed to have 90% power.

An important assumption when using historical data is that of consistency. The true treatment effect must be consistent in the historical and current data. If this assumption is not valid, results may be biased and yield higher rates of false-positive (type I) and false-negative (type II) errors. In the above example, if the true drug effect is really 0, but the prior data suggestive of a drug effect are incorporated, the probability of a false-positive result is 19%, compared to the 5% rate in the traditional method.

This example illustrates the previously noted point that use of historical data involves a trade-off between bias and precision. Given the context here is comparison vs. SoC, historical data will likely be abundant since standards of care are well-studied. Therefore, it may be useful to select subsets of the historical data that most closely match the situation at hand in order to ensure validity of the consistency assumption.

It may also be useful to consider adaptive designs (Chow and Chang, 2007). For example, in a Bayesian augmented design, patients could be randomized to placebo, test drug, and SoC, with an interim analysis conducted when the test drug versus placebo contrast is adequately powered. If the interim result is positive, enrollment continues until the test drug versus SoC contrast is sufficiently reliable, including an appropriate set of historical data as an informative prior in a Bayesian analysis.

Portfolio modeling and simulation

The fundamental premise of a portfolio perspective on clinical trial design is that optimizing each individual trial in a series of trials does not necessarily optimize the series of trials. By extension, optimizing each in a series of compounds does not necessarily optimize the portfolio of compounds. Sophisticated simulations of virtual compounds and portfolios are needed to simultaneously consider the many factors that might influence the characteristics of studies needed to optimize the portfolio and the designs to achieve those characteristics. Nevertheless, simple examples can illustrate how modeling and simulation of portfolios of drugs can influence the designs for individual trials.

Consider a portfolio of 100 drugs to be tested in PoC studies. One of the most straight-forward questions to ask about an individual PoC study is what level of power and type I error is desired. The interrelationships between probability of efficacy [p(E)], power, and type I error rate on the number of launches (drugs receiving regulatory approval) are summarized in Table 7 and illustrated in Figure 1.

The rate of false-positive results is half the type I error rate (when using a two-tailed test), and the false-negative rate is 1 – power. Consider rows 6 and 8 in Table 7. The sample sizes are approximately equal for these two scenarios. With p(E) = 20% (20 of the 100 compounds are effective) using 90% power with a false-positive rate of 5% (row 8) yields 18 launches and four Phase III failures, whereas 80% power with a false positive rate of 2.5% (row 6) yields 16 launches and two Phase III failures. If the profit from a launch exceeds the cost of a Phase III failure then the 90% power scenario would be more profitable.

A number of other useful comparisons arise from the table. Comparing results within blocks of three (1–3, 4–6, 7–9, 10–12, 13–15, 16–18) illustrates the influence of the rate of false-positive findings. Comparing the following sets of rows isolates the impact of power: (1, 4, 7) (2, 5, 8) (3, 6, 9) (10, 13, 16) (11, 14, 17) (12, 15, 18). Comparing the following sets of rows isolates the impact of p(E): (1, 10) (2, 11) (3, 12), etc.

Figure 1 further illustrates the effect of Phase II power and alpha on the portfolio at a fixed p(E)=20%. As power increases and alpha level decreases in Phase II (Figure 1a), the percent of successful Phase III studies increases. However, this benefit is offset by increasing Phase II costs (Figure 1b); the Phase II sample size must increase to achieve the desired higher power and lower alpha level. Therefore, due to budgetary constraints, the differential cost of successful launches versus Phase III failures, the market value of each molecule, cycle time, and other factors, a trade-off is needed to determine the optimal Phase II operating characteristics for a given scenario.

General conclusions from these comparisons include that control of false-positive results in PoC studies influences the Phase III success rate – the efficiency of the portfolio. Power influences the number of launches – the effectiveness of the portfolio. And p(E) influences both efficiency and effectiveness. However, the interrelationships between these factors are also important. For example, the false-positive rate has a greater influence when p(E) is lower as the need for protection against false-positive results increases as the percent of effective drugs decreases. Similarly, power has a greater influence when p(E) is higher as the need for protection against false-negative results increases as the percent of effective drugs increases.

From the example it might be tempting to conclude that high power and low rates of false positive results in PoC studies are optimal. However, to illustrate points, a number of simplifying assumptions have been made, most notably, that of studying a fixed portfolio of 100 drugs with unlimited resources. An alternative example where the budget is fixed and the number of potential drugs to investigate is unlimited, or at least greater than the budget allows, can be constructed to show that smaller studies with lower power and higher rates of false-positive results are optimal because the smaller sample sizes facilitate study of more drugs, which in turn results in more launches.

Therefore, the point of this example is not to lobby for one approach or another. Rather the intent is to illustrate that a portfolio perspective can influence development strategies, which in turn can – and should – influence the design of individual clinical trials.

Placebo response and signal detection

Signal detection is the term often used to describe the ability to differentiate between an effective drug and placebo; that is, to find a treatment effect when one exists (Mallinckrodt

Table 7. Attributes of a Phase III portfolio resulting from a Phase II portfolio of 100 drugs across varying levels; the number of effective drugs, power, and type I error rate

Row	p(E)	Power	False pos rate	n per arm	True positives	False positives	Total positive	True negatives	False negatives	Total negatives	Phase III portfolio	Phase III success	Launches
1	20	0.65	0.1	35	13	8	21	72	7	79	21	61.9%	13
2	20	0.65	0.05	52	13	4	17	76	7	83	17	76.5%	13
3	20	0.65	0.025	69	13	2	15	78	7	85	15	86.7%	13
4	20	0.8	0.1	57	16	8	24	72	4	76	24	66.7%	16
5	20	0.8	0.05	78	16	4	20	76	4	80	20	80.0%	16
6	20	0.8	0.025	99	16	2	18	78	4	82	18	88.9%	16
7	20	0.9	0.1	83	18	8	26	72	2	74	26	69.2%	18
8	20	0.9	0.05	108	18	4	22	76	2	78	22	81.8%	18
9	20	0.9	0.025	132	18	2	20	78	2	80	20	90.0%	18
10	30	0.65	0.1	35	19.5	7	26.5	63	10.5	73.5	26.5	73.6%	19.5
11	30	0.65	0.05	52	19.5	3.5	23	66.5	10.5	77	23	84.8%	19.5
12	30	0.65	0.025	69	19.5	1.75	21.25	68.25	10.5	78.75	21.25	91.8%	19.5
13	30	0.8	0.1	57	24	7	31	63	6	69	31	77.4%	24
14	30	0.8	0.05	78	24	3.5	27.5	66.5	6	72.5	27.5	87.3%	24
15	30	0.8	0.025	99	24	1.75	25.75	68.25	6	74.25	25.75	93.2%	24
16	30	0.9	0.1	83	27	7	34	63	3	66	34	79.4%	27
17	30	0.9	0.05	108	27	3.5	30.5	66.5	3	69.5	30.5	88.5%	27
18	30	0.9	0.025	132	27	1.75	28.75	68.25	3	71.25	28.75	93.9%	27

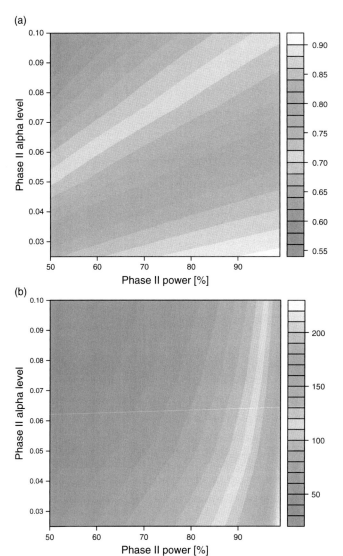

(a)

(b)

Figure 1. (a) Colormap of the Phase III success rate versus the Phase II power and alpha level when p(E)=0.2. (b) Colormap of the sample size per arm needed in a Phase II study versus power and alpha level for p(E)=0.2. See plate section for color version.

et al., 2007). Among the CNS diseases, perhaps the most research on placebo response and signal detection has been in major depressive disorder (MDD). Khan *et al.* (2003) found that placebo response was strongly associated with the ability to differentiate an effective antidepressant from placebo. They reported that when using a mean change from baseline of 30% to dichotomize trials as having high or low placebo response, the proportion of contrasts from effective drugs that showed significant differences from placebo was 21.1% in trials with high placebo response and 74.2% in trials with low placebo response.

Observational and causal components

Yang *et al.* (2005) provide a useful summary of the many papers on the causes and potential cures for high placebo response. They define placebo response as the change that occurs

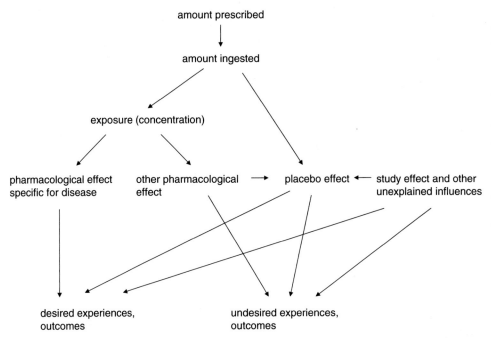

Figure 2. Diagram of outcomes and their causal pathways.

after administration of placebo, with total placebo response being attributable to a study effect plus a placebo effect. The study effect includes such factors as spontaneous improvement, regression to the mean, improvement due to superior care provided in the trial as compared to the treatment received prior to trial participation, etc. The study effect could be assessed as the change in patients participating in the trial who were not administered a medication. The authors further define the placebo effect as the difference between placebo response (the response in placebo-treated patients) and the study effect. The active drug effect is defined as that portion of the overall response in drug-treated patients due to the pharmacodynamic properties of the drug, which can be assessed as the difference in response between drug-treated and placebo-treated patients.

A diagram of the various influences on outcomes is depicted in Figure 2. Study medication can produce desired and undesired effects. However, placebo can also produce desired and undesired effects directly as a result of patient expectation. Placebo effects can also be produced indirectly through other pharmacological effects of the drug that convince patients they are not on placebo. Moreover, placebo effects can be enhanced via study effects helping to convince patients that the study medication is working. The main message from this diagram is that the placebo effect and placebo response is complex, with many potential causes leading to a variety of outcomes.

Controlling placebo response

Therefore, it is not surprising that as Yang *et al.* (2005) summarize, a wide array of factors have been associated with placebo response and trial outcome. But results have been

Evolution of Antidepressants

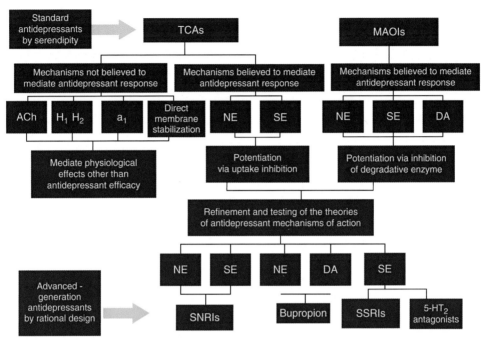

Figure 1.2 From TCAs and MAOIs to newer antidepressants.

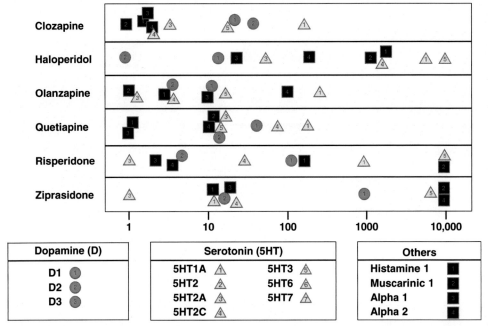

Figure 1.3 Comparison of the binding affinity of chlorpromazine, haloperidol and newer "atypical" antipsychotics. The profile for each drug is expressed relative to its most potent binding.

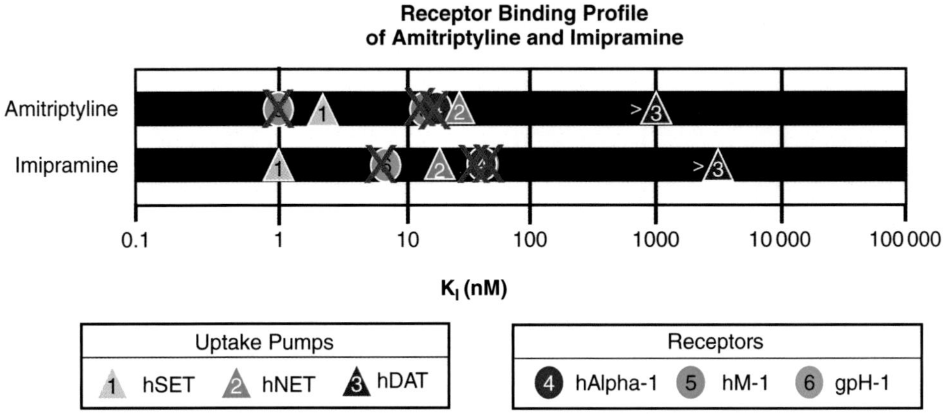

Figure 1.4 Receptor binding profile of TCAs.

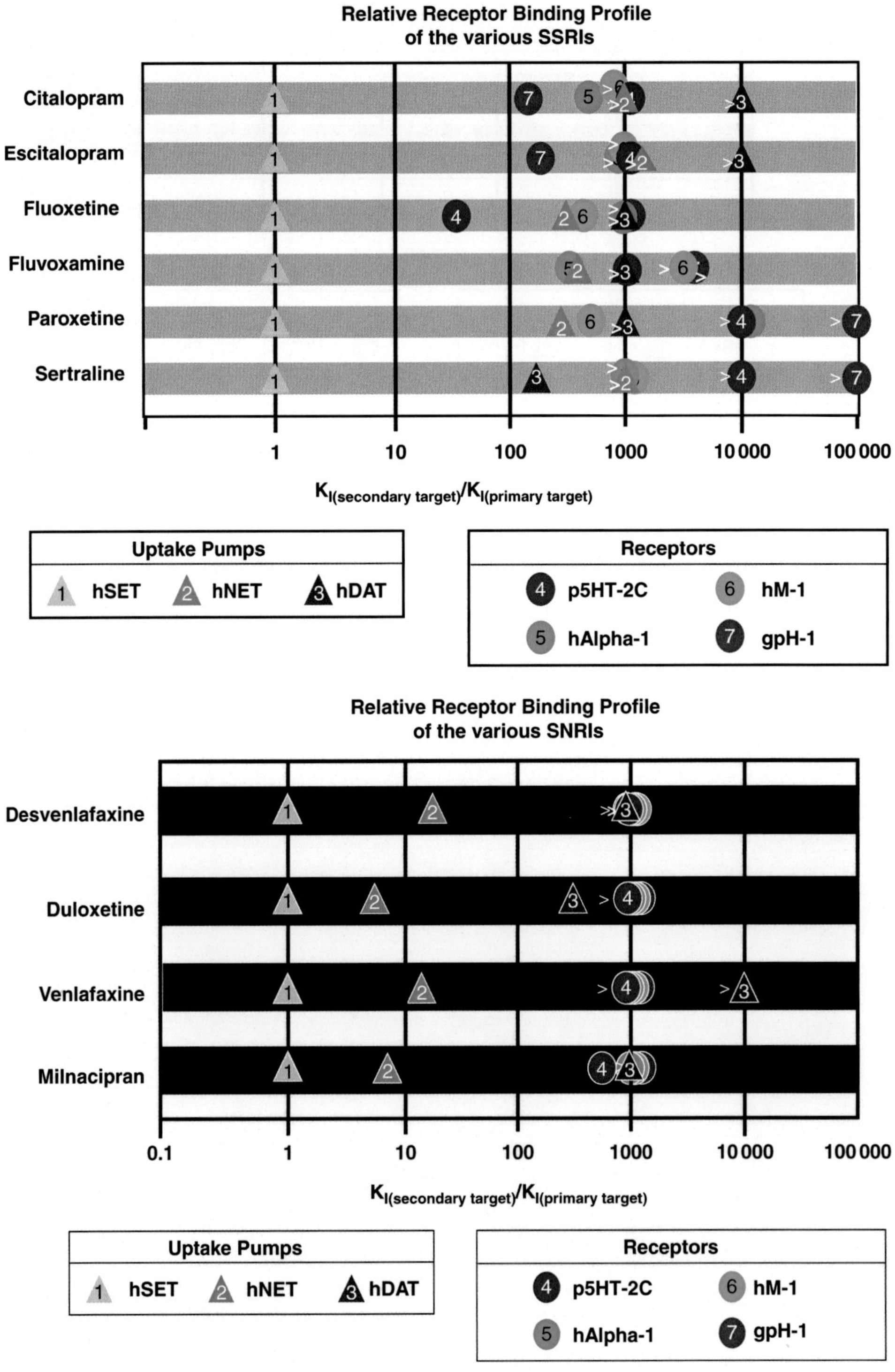

Figure 1.5 Comparison of the relative receptor binding profile of SSRIs and SNRIs.

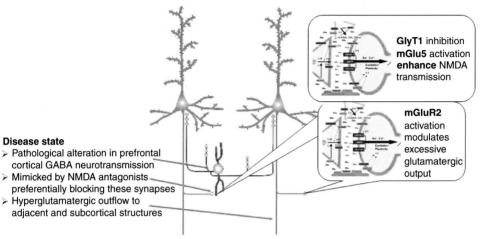

Schizophrenia

- Schematic of Glutamate Hypothesis

GlyT1 inhibition
mGlu5 activation
enhance NMDA
transmission

mGluR2
activation
modulates
excessive
glutamatergic
output

Disease state
➤ Pathological alteration in prefrontal
cortical GABA neurotransmission
➤ Mimicked by NMDA antagonists
preferentially blocking these synapses
➤ Hyperglutamatergic outflow to
adjacent and subcortical structures

Symptom clusters reflect divergent output pathways

| ➤ Hippocampus | ➤ Cortical association pathways | ➤ Midbrain dopamine |
| • Working memory | • Executive function | • Psychosis |

Figure 3.6 Systems-based approach to drug discovery in psychiatry.

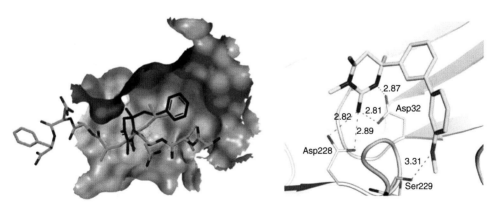

Figure 3.8 Fragment-based approaches to lead generation.

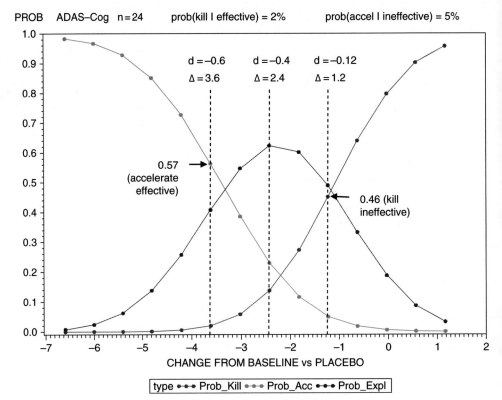

Figure 5.2 In this example of a first, small efficacy study in Alzheimer's disease, the desired drug-placebo difference (effective drug) on the ADAS-cog outcome measure is 3.6 points (effect size −0.6). A drug-placebo difference of 1.2 (or less) is clearly unacceptable (ineffective). The acceptable probability of advancing an ineffective drug is set at 5%, and the acceptable probability of stopping an effective drug is set at 2%. Given the variability of the ADAS-cog (standard deviation = 6), if the true effect of the drug candidate is 3.6 points, with a sample size of 24 in a 2 x 2 crossover design, there is a 57% probability of advancing an effective drug candidate, a 41% chance of ending up uncertain, and a 2% chance of stopping an effective drug candidate. The probability of stopping an ineffective drug candidate (true drug-placebo difference 1.2 points) is 46%, the probability of ending up uncertain is 49%, and the probability of advancing an ineffective drug candidate is 5%. One can create and examine similar graphical displays for various sample sizes, setting various acceptable probabilities for advancing an ineffective drug or stopping and effective drug, to facilitate getting agreement on the decision rules for the study and to determine the size of investment to make. Probabilities for correct and incorrect decision-making for true drug effects between 1.2 and 3.6 points can also be determined (e.g. 2.4 points is shown).

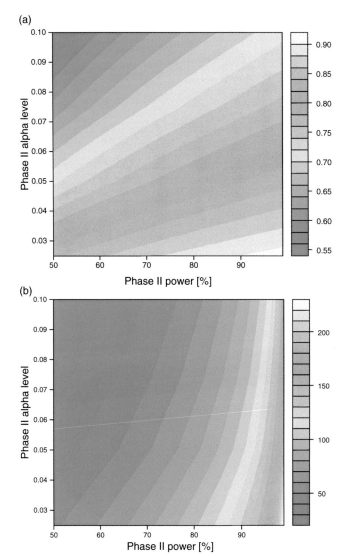

Figure 7.1 (a) Colormap of the Phase III success rate versus the Phase II power and alpha level when p(E)=0.2. (b) Colormap of the sample size per arm needed in a Phase II study versus power and alpha level for p(E)=0.2.

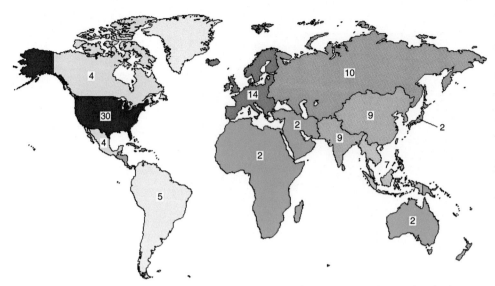

Figure 8.1 Clinical trial research activity in schizophrenia. Number of trials per region. Source: clinicaltrials.gov, Dec. 2009.

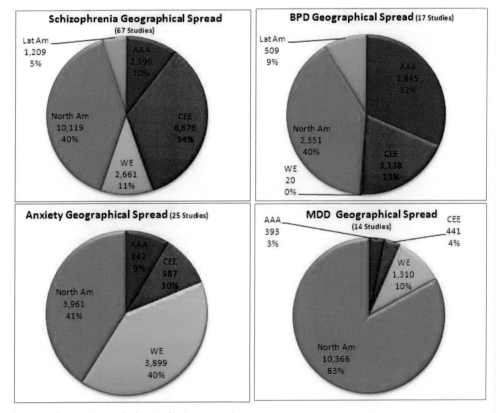

Figure 8.3 Patients recruited per indication per region.

inconsistent, owing in part to the inherent limitations of these predominantly retrospective studies. And even those factors that have consistently been associated with trial outcome in retrospective analyses may not result in improved drug-placebo discrimination when implemented prospectively.

Consider for example baseline severity. Even if having more severely ill patients curbed placebo response and improved signal detection, the more restrictive entry criteria slow enrollment. In practice, much of the benefit from the restricted population may be lost if pressure to enroll is great, thereby increasing the tendency for baseline score inflation (Landin et al., 2000). Therefore, despite a long-standing focus on placebo response in MDD, solutions have proven elusive (Walsh et al., 2002). And placebo response is becoming a serious problem in disease states where it has not formerly been problematic. For example, a recent report for schizophrenia noted that placebo response was increasing at an alarming rate, and signal detection was becoming more difficult (Kemp et al., 2008).

Further, an increasing body of literature is pointing to patient expectation as having a key role in placebo response (Rutherford et al., 2009). For example, the likelihood a patient will receive an effective drug versus receiving placebo has been hypothesized to influence expectation of improvement and in turn placebo response (Papakostas and Fava, 2009). The authors therefore hypothesized that the percentage of patients randomized to placebo should be associated with placebo response. They tested this hypothesis via a meta-analysis of 182 clinical trials in depression, involving 262 treatment arm contrasts with placebo. A multivariate regression analysis was used to assess the independent effects of several predictors. The factor that had the greatest influence on drug-placebo differences was the percentage of patients randomized to placebo. As the percent randomized to placebo increased, drug-placebo differences increased. Using the results of this study, Table 8 summarizes the expected difference between drug and placebo in response rates across various common percentages of patients randomized to placebo. When 50% of patients are randomized to placebo the advantage of drug over placebo is expected to be 50% larger (18% vs. 12%) than when 25% of patients are randomized to placebo.

From a statistical theory perspective, there is no mechanism through which the probability of allocation to placebo or number of treatment arms can influence treatment contrasts. However, for fixed total sample size, as the number of treatment arms increases, the variance of each treatment arm contrast is minimized, and therefore the probability of getting at least one significant drug-placebo contrast is maximized, when the placebo group has greater allocation than the individual treatment arms.

Specifically, for studies with two, three, and four active treatment arms, the maximum probability of at least one significant drug-placebo contrast is achieved with 41.4%, 36.6%, and 33.3% of patients randomized to placebo, respectively. The basis for this can be appreciated by considering a trial with equal allocation. If one patient is added to the placebo group the power for all drug-placebo contrasts is increased, whereas if one patient is added to an active treatment arm that is the only contrast where power is increased.

Nearly optimal allocation ratios to maximize power for a series of pairwise contrasts with a control can be obtained with practical randomization schemes. For example, in a three-arm study allocation of patients to placebo and the two drug arms in a 4:3:3 ratio yields 40% on placebo, which is close to the optimum 41.4%. Similarly, for a four-arm study allocation of 3:2:2:2 yields 33.3% on placebo and is close to the optimal 36.3%. And for a five-arm study allocation of 2:1:1:1:1 yields the optimal ratio with 33.3% randomized to placebo.

Table 8. Percent of patients randomized to placebo and expected drug–placebo differences in response rate for clinical trials in major depressive disorder

% randomized to placebo	Drug–placebo difference in response rates (%)
20	11
25	12
33.3	14
50	18

This discussion assumes that the focus is on a series of pairwise contrasts versus control. Such a perspective may be more common in confirmatory trials and less common in earlier-phase studies where a variety of methods for assessing dose response may be employed. Therefore, increasing the probability of allocation to placebo may not increase power in all situations and should be evaluated in each circumstance. Moreover, it is not known if the results seen in MDD regarding placebo allocation apply more broadly across CNS disorders.

Other means of improving signal detection

While placebo response has an important influence on signal detection, it is not the only factor. For example, core factor subscales have been shown to yield larger effect sizes than the total score of the Hamilton Depression Rating Scale (Mallinckrodt *et al.*, 2007). And the MMRM (Mixed-effects Model for Repeated Measures) analytic approach provides better control of false-positive and false-negative results than last observation carried forward (LOCF) (Mallinckrodt *et al.*, 2008), and thereby has improved signal detection in depression clinical trials (Mallinckrodt *et al.*, 2007).

Table 9 summarizes differences in outcome by method of analysis, percent randomized to placebo, and total scores vs. subscales for contrasts of a test drug and active comparators with placebo during the development of an antidepressant.

Given the complexities of placebo response, no single strategy can solve the problem. However, starting with optimum designs and analysis may provide important benefits in their own right and may have additional benefits in other areas. For example, by improving signal detection via design and analysis, sample size can be reduced. This reduction may facilitate use of fewer investigative sites and/or the ability to restrict patient selection in ways that might further improve signal detection.

Missing data and data analysis

Many clinical trials in CNS disorders use a design wherein patients are assessed repeatedly over time. Although the contrast between treatments at a specific time, such as the endpoint assessment, is often the primary focus, interest also exists in the trends over time. Verbeke and Molenberghs (2000) provide a detailed and broad review of the longitudinal data analyses relevant in such settings.

Table 9. Average effect sizes for test drug and active comparators by method of analysis, outcome measure, and percent randomized to placebo from the duloxetine development program in major depressive disorder

Design	Analysis	Endpoint	Effect size
All studies	LOCF	HAMD total	.294[1]
All studies	MMRM	HAMD total	.384[1]
All studies	MMRM	Maier subscale	.452[1]
Studies with 50% randomized to placebo	MMRM	Maier subscale	.635[2]

[1]Mallinckrodt *et al.* 2007.
[2]Data on file LRL.
Table reused with permission from *Drug Information Journal.*

One issue of particular importance in the analysis of CNS clinical trials is missing data. Dropout rates in CNS trials are frequently over 30% (Khan *et al.*, 2007). Such high rates of missing data are concerning because of the increased likelihood of bias and the associated likelihood that the method used to handle the missing data will influence results and inferences drawn from them.

Theory

There is no universally best approach for longitudinal analyses. In order to understand the potential impact of missing data and to choose an appropriate method for a particular situation, the process (i.e. mechanisms) leading to the missingness must be considered. The following taxonomy of missing-data mechanisms is now well-established in the statistical literature (Little and Rubin, 1987).

Data are *missing completely at random* (MCAR) if, conditional upon the independent variables in the analytic model, the probability of missingness does not depend on either the observed or unobserved outcomes of the variable being analyzed (dependent variable). Data are *missing at random* (MAR) if, conditional upon the independent variables in the analytic model and the observed outcomes of the dependent variable, the probability of missingness does not depend on the unobserved outcomes of the dependent variable. Data are *missing not at random* (MNAR) if, conditional upon the independent variables in the analytic model and the observed outcomes of the dependent variable, the probability of missingness *does* depend on the unobserved outcomes of the variable being analyzed.

Several key points arise from these definitions. First, the characterization of the missingness mechanism does not rest on the data alone; it involves both the data and the model used to analyze them. Consequently, missingness that might be MNAR given one model could be MAR or MCAR given another. In addition, since the relationship between the dependent variable and missingness is a key factor in the missingness mechanism, the mechanism may vary from one outcome to the next within the same data set.

Moreover, when drop-out rates differ by treatment group, it would be incorrect to conclude that the missingness mechanism giving rise to the drop-out is MNAR and that analyses assuming MCAR or MAR would be invalid. If drop-out depends only on treatment, and treatment is included in the analytic model, the mechanism giving rise to the drop-out would be MCAR. It is also important to realize that when some data are missing all analyses rely on assumptions about the mechanism giving rise to the missingness (Mallinckrodt *et al.*, 2008).

Analyses

Historically, single imputation methods such as last (and baseline) observation carried forward (LOCF, BOCF) were common methods of handling missing data in CNS drug development. These methods require restrictive assumptions, such as MCAR and others. But they were initially useful due to ease of implementation in an era when computing resources were limited and statistical theory on missing data was only emerging.

Advances in computing power and the development of software tools allowed researchers to routinely implement methods valid under the less restrictive assumption of MAR (Mallinckrodt *et al.*, 2008; Molenberghs and Kenward, 2007). The MAR assumption is often reasonable in longitudinal clinical trials. At a minimum, MAR is more plausible than MCAR because MAR is always valid if MCAR is valid, but MAR is valid in cases when MCAR is not (Mallinckrodt *et al.*, 2008; Molenberghs and Kenward, 2007; Verbeke and Molenberghs, 2000). Moreover, it has been unequivocally established that MAR methods provide better control of Type I and Type II error than LOCF and BOCF regardless of whether the missingness mechanism is MAR or MNAR (Mallinckrodt *et al.*, 2008; Siddiqui *et al.*, 2009).

Analyses valid under MAR that have been commonly used in CNS clinical trials include the mixed-effects model for repeated measures, or so-called MMRM approach. MMRM is a specific member from the broader class of direct likelihood-based analyses (Mallinckrodt *et al.*, 2008). Another analytic method valid under MAR that is widely applicable to CNS clinical trials is multiple imputation.

Although MAR is often reasonable, the possibility of MNAR data resulting in meaningful bias to estimates of treatment effects from an MAR analysis is impossible to rule out. Therefore, analyses valid under MNAR are needed. When MAR is not valid, the observed data are not a valid predictor of the unobserved data. The fundamental difficulty in MNAR analyses is that going beyond MAR, beyond what the observed data predict, can only be done via assumptions about the unobserved data. Therefore, conclusions from MNAR analyses are conditional on the appropriateness of the assumed model. But these assumptions are not testable, because we do not have the missing data for which the assumptions are made (Laird, 1994).

Hence, no individual MNAR analysis can be considered definitive. Not surprisingly then, many statistical methodologies have been proposed to analyze data in the MNAR setting. General classes of MNAR methods have arisen from different factorizations of the likelihood functions for the joint distribution of the outcome variable and the indicator variable for whether or not a data point is observed. Factorization in this context means that the hypothetical "full" data are split into two parts: the actually observed part and the missing part, which are often described as the measurement process and the missingness process, respectively (Molenberghs and Kenward, 2007; Verbeke and Molenberghs, 2000).

While the technical details of these various methods are important to statisticians, the key point is that various MNAR methods are built on different assumptions. Therefore, implementing a series of MNAR analyses fosters an understanding of how sensitive results are to assumptions about the missing data. In other words, they are ideally suited for implementation in a sensitivity analysis framework (Molenberghs and Kenward, 2007; Verbeke and Molenberghs, 2000).

Another approach to sensitivity analyses is what Collins *et al.* (2001) referred to as inclusive modeling, which is done within the MAR framework. Restrictive models that are typical of primary analyses include as independent variables only the design variables of the study, such as treatment, time, investigative site, with baseline severity and its interaction with time as covariates. In addition to the design factors, inclusive models add "ancillary variables" to the analysis. The basic idea stems from the definition of MAR: conditional upon the variables in the model, missingness does not depend on the unobserved outcomes of the variable being analyzed. Therefore, if additional (ancillary) variables are added to the model that help explain missingness, MAR can be valid, whereas if the additional variables were not included the data would be MNAR.

Multiple imputation is well suited for inclusive modeling. With separate steps for imputation and analysis, ancillary variables that are post-baseline, time-varying covariates – possibly influenced by treatment – can be included in the imputation step but then not included in the analysis step. This approach can avoid the confounding of the treatment effects on the response variable with post-baseline covariates that are also influenced by treatment, as might be the case in a likelihood-based analysis.

The widespread use of LOCF and BOCF set historical precedent that fostered their continued acceptance even as advancements in statistical theory and in our ability to implement the theory might have otherwise relegated them to the museum of statistics. LOCF and BOCF are still used in drug development, primarily based on their intuitive appeal as measures of effectiveness; that is, as a composite of efficacy, safety, and tolerability. For a comprehensive review of the varying perspectives on missing data an entire issue of *Drug Information Journal* (Volume 43, Number 4, July 2009) has been devoted to the topic.

Literally taken, LOCF and BOCF imply imputation of missing values at specific time points – a longitudinal context. However, an alternative interpretation of LOCF is commonly used that might be better termed LO (last observation). In this approach, results are interpreted as the change that was actually seen at last observation regardless of when it was observed – an effectiveness context. With BOCF, a similar interpretation may be used. However, rather than using the last observation, the baseline value is used assuming that patients who discontinue drug received no lasting benefit. Numerically, results from the longitudinal and effectiveness contexts are identical. It is only the interpretation that differs.

While these non-longitudinal interpretations of LOCF and BOCF may be intuitively appealing, that does not guarantee meaningful results. For example, LOCF and BOCF can in some situations yield smaller estimates of treatment differences when patients drop out due to adverse events; the reduction is not necessarily proportional to the safety risk. In addition, drop-out may be occurring for many reasons, some associated with risk, some not. Moreover, LOCF and BOCF are known to inflate false-positive and false-negative rates, which will be the case regardless of whether results are interpreted in the longitudinal or effectiveness context (Mallinckrodt *et al.*, 2008; Mallinckrodt and Kenward, 2009).

Perhaps most importantly, the analysis must be matched with the design. The primary purpose of clinical trials is typically to delineate differences between drug and control that are attributable to the drug. Double-blind randomized designs are appropriate for these causal inferences. However, it is unreasonable to assume that doctors and patients make the

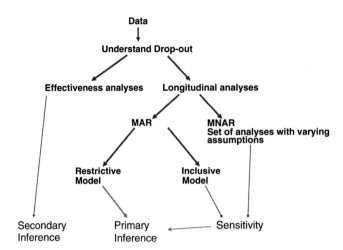

Figure 3. Analytic road map for continuous endpoints in longitudinal clinical trials.

same decisions regarding continuation of therapy in a double-blind trial, in which they are unsure about whether the patient is taking drug or placebo, as they would make in actual practice, when the drug and its properties are well known. Therefore, the rates and reasons for drop-out within the strictly controlled conditions of a confirmatory clinical trial are unlikely to mirror what would happen in general use.

When effectiveness is the primary objective, the best place to assess it would be in a general medical (i.e. naturalistic) setting. Hence, using LOCF or BOCF in an effectiveness context is inconsistent with the design and primary objective of confirmatory clinical trials (Mallinckrodt *et al.*, 2008; Mallinckrodt and Kenward, 2009).

Analytic road map

Broad consensus has emerged indicating that the primary analyses of longitudinal clinical trials with continuous endpoints should be based on MAR (Mallinckrodt *et al.*, 2008; Molenberghs and Kenward, 2007; Siddiqui *et al.*, 2009; Verbeke and Molenberghs, 2000). In many circumstances, the primary analysis will be based on a restrictive model. For sensitivity analyses, a variety of MNAR methods based on differing assumptions can be implemented along with MAR methods using inclusive models. Effectiveness analyses can be conducted secondarily using LOCF, BOCF, or other means. This analytic road map is illustrated in Figure 3.

Concluding remarks

In this chapter, design decisions were approached from an over-arching framework that defines development strategies as fast to PoC, or fast to registration. Choices of these primary archetypes are driven by the axes of development: optimism for success and signal detection. Secondary archetypes are used to mitigate trade-offs between the primary archetypes, thereby optimizing development. Adaptive designs were discussed as a means to mitigate trade-offs between the primary archetypes. Adaptive designs and Bayesian approaches were discussed as means to more efficiently facilitate early comparisons between a test drug and SoC. Conditions under which use of a positive control might be beneficial were identified. Throughout the chapter, simple examples were used to illustrate individual concepts on how a portfolio perspective can optimize the design of individual clinical trials, the development plans of individual compounds, and the development of entire portfolios. Portfolio modeling and simulation were introduced as a means to move from simplistic examples of individual concepts to sophisticated integration of many factors for portfolio optimization.

Although adaptive designs, Bayesian methods, and modeling and simulation hold promise for improving CNS drug development, rigor must continue to be placed on the long-standing problems of missing data and placebo response. Here too, progress has been made, but this progress cannot be taken for granted and continued vigilance and research is required.

Literally hundreds of books and thousands of papers have been written on statistical principles related to the design and analysis of clinical trials. Thus, many of these principles are well-known. Yet, drug development becomes ever more challenging. Perhaps the difficulties lay not as much in knowing the principles, but rather in putting them into useful practice. If so, hopefully a portfolio perspective will be beneficial in applying the principles more effectively.

References

Berry, D. A. and Stangl, D. K. (Eds.) (1996). *Bayesian Biostatistics*. New York: Marcel Dekker.

Chow, S.-C. and Chang, M. (2007). *Adaptive Design Methods in Clinical Trials*. Boca Raton, FL: Chapman and Hall/CRC.

Collins, L. M., Schafer, J. L., and Kam, C. M. (2001). A comparison of inclusive and restrictive strategies in modern missing data procedures. *Psychol Methods*, 6 (4), 330–51.

Gallo, P., Chuang-Stein, C., Dragalin, V., *et al.* (2006). Adaptive designs in clinical drug development – an executive summary of the PhRMA Working Group. *J Biopharmaceut Stat*, 16, 275–83.

Hurko, O. and Ryan, J. L. (2005). Translational research in central nervous system drug discovery. *NeuroRx*, 2, 671–82.

ICH guidelines; E4: Dose-response information to support drug registration; E8: General considerations for clinical trials. Accessed at http://www.ich.org/cache/compo/276-254-1.

Kemp, A. S., Schooler, N. R., Kalali, A. H., *et al.* (2008). What is causing the reduced drug-placebo difference in recent schizophrenia clinical trials and what can be done about it? *Schizophr Bull*, doi:10.1093/schbul/sbn110.

Khan, A., Detke, M., Khan, S. R., and Mallinckrodt, C. (2003). Placebo response and antidepressant clinical trial outcome. *J Nerv Ment Dis*, 191, 211–18.

Khan, A., Schwartz, K., Redding, N., Kolts, R., and Brown, W. (2007). Psychiatric and Clinical Trial Completion Rates: Diagnosis analysis of the FDA SBA reports. *Neuropsychopharmacology*, 32, 2422–30.

Kola, I. and Landis, J. (2004). Can the pharmaceutical industry reduce attrition rates? *Nat Rev Drug Discov*, 3, 711–15.

Laird, N. M. (1994). Discussion to Diggle, P. J., Kenward, M. G. Informative dropout in longitudinal data analysis. *Appl Stat*, 43, 84.

Landin, R., DeBrota, D. J., DeVries, T. A., Potter, W. Z., and Demitrack, M. A. (2000). The impact of restrictive entry criterion during the placebo lead-in period. *Biometrics*, 56, 271–8.

Lieberman, J. A., Greenhouse, J., Hamer, R. M., *et al.* (2005). Comparing the effects of antidepressants: consensus guidelines for evaluating quantitative reviews of antidepressant efficacy. *Neuropsychopharmacology*, 30, 445–60.

Little, R. and Rubin, D. (1987). *Statistical Analysis with Missing Data*. New York: John Wiley & Sons.

Mallinckrodt, C. H., Meyers, A. L., Prakash, A., Faries, D. E., and Detke, M. J. (2007). Simple options for improving signal detection in antidepressant clinical trials. *Psychopharmacol Bull*, 40, 101–14.

Mallinckrodt, C. H., Lane, P. W., Schnell, D., Peng, Y., and Mancuso, J. P. (2008). Recommendations for the primary analysis of continuous endpoints in longitudinal clinical trials. *Drug Inf J*, 42, 305–19.

Mallinckrodt, C. H. and Kenward, M. G. (2009). Conceptual considerations regarding endpoints, hypotheses, and analyses for incomplete longitudinal clinical trial data. *Drug Inf J*, 43, 449–58.

Mallinckrodt, C. H., Detke, M. J., Prucka, W. R., Ruberg, S. J., and Molenberghs, G. (2010a). Design archetypes for Phase II clinical trials in central nervous system disorders. *Drug Inf J*. Accepted.

Mallinckrodt, C. H., Detke, M. J., Prucka, W. R., Ruberg, S. J., and Molenberghs, G. (2010b). Considerations for using positive controls in Phase II clinical trials of central nervous system disorders. *Drug Inf J*. Accepted.

Mallinckrodt, C. H., Detke, M. J., Prucka, W. R., Ruberg, S. J., and Molenberghs, G. (2010c). Considerations for comparing a test drug with standard of care in Phase II clinical trials of central nervous system disorders. *Drug Inf J*. Accepted.

Molenberghs, G. and Kenward, M. G. (2007). *Missing Data in Clinical Studies*. Chichester: John Wiley & Sons.

Papakostas, G. I. and Fava, M. (2009). Does the probability of receiving placebo influence clinical trial outcome? A meta-regression of double-blind, randomized clinical trials in MDD. *Eur Neuropsychopharmacol*, 19, 34–40.

Piantadosi, S. (2005). *Clinical Trials: A Methodologic Perspective*. Hoboken, NJ: John Wiley & Sons.

Rutherford, B. R., Rose, S. A., Sneed, J. R., and Roose, S. P. (2009). Study design affects participant expectations: a survey. *J Clin Psychopharmacol*, 29, 179–81.

Siddiqui, O., Hung, H. M., and O'Neill, R. O. (2009). MMRM vs. LOCF: a comprehensive comparison based on simulation study and 25 NDA datasets. *J Biopharmaceut Stat*, 19 (2), 227–46.

Spiegelhalter, D. J., Abrams, K. R., and Myles, J. P. (2004). *Bayesian Approaches to Clinical Trials and Health-Care Evaluation*. New York: John Wiley & Sons.

Temple, R. and Ellenberg, S. S. (2000). Placebo-controlled trials and active-control trials in the evaluation of new treatments. Part 1: ethical and scientific issues. *Ann Intern Med*, 133 (6), 455–63.

Verbeke, G. and Molenberghs, G. (2000). *Linear Mixed Models for Longitudinal Data*. New York: Springer.

Walsh, B. T., Seidman, S. N., Sysko, R., and Gould, M. (2002). Placebo response in studies of major depression: variable, substantial, and growing. *J Am Med Assoc*, 287, 1840–7.

Yang, H., Cusin, C., and Fava, M. (2005). Is there a problem in antidepressant trials? *Curr Top Med Chem*, 5, 1077–86.

Clinical trials management at company level

Nuala Murphy

Introduction

The greatest challenge in clinical development in the field of psychiatry is the risk of failure. The literature indicates that many multiple randomized clinical trials in depression, anxiety, and schizophrenia have failed to demonstrate a drug effect with as many as 60% of depression trials being reported as failed trials (Andrews, 2001; Antonuccio *et al.*, 2002; Brown, 1995; Forest Laboratories, 1998; Ker *et al.*, 2000; Kirby *et al.*, 2005; Kirsch *et al.*, 2002; Lane, 1999; Laughren, 1998; Lipton, 2000; Oosterbaan *et al.*, 2001). Such a high failure rate results in the loss of millions of dollars and the failure of many compounds to advance to market. A number of reasons have been advanced to explain this observation, including subject and site interactions, trial design, site–sponsor interactions, rating scale deficiencies, and trial management, i.e. speed of recruitment and inadequate diagnosis (Kirsch *et al.*, 2002). Furthermore, clinical trials have been shown to take 42% longer than expected to complete in Phase I, 31% longer in Phase II, and 30% beyond planned deadlines in Phase III (Cutting Edge Information, 2004) resulting also in major financial losses and missed NDA deadlines.

With this in mind, the current chapter aims to address the key elements of CNS trial management required to drive successful outcomes in a high-risk environment. The objective of CNS trial management is to ensure that protocols are feasible, patients are eligible, the trial is conducted according to ICH-GCP guidelines, and finally that conclusive data are provided in a timely and cost-effective manner. Where studies in psychiatry are concerned, the real challenge for management is related to the subjective nature of the data required to demonstrate efficacy. This chapter will address how each of these topics may influence study conduct.

In the past decade, the majority of trials in psychiatry have been conducted in schizophrenia, bipolar disorder, major depressive disorder, and generalized anxiety disorder and to this end will be the key indications discussed in this chapter.

A case study

In support of this chapter, an analysis of 123 studies conducted globally in schizophrenia, bipolar disorder, major depressive disorder, and generalized anxiety disorder has been performed. Key aspects of trial management such as:

Essential CNS Drug Development, ed. A. Kalali, Sheldon Preskorn, J. Kwentus, and Stephen M. Stahl. Published by Cambridge University Press. © Cambridge University Press 2012.

- country acceptance of placebo-controlled trials
- timelines for approval
- site experience
- patient access and accrual experience
- pitfalls in meeting timelines
- contingency planning

have been drawn from the experience acquired not only at the regulatory level but at the operational level globally. Details on the geographic contribution and source of data are provided in Appendix 1.

Regulatory guidance

When designing clinical development plans, guidance should be sought from the European Agency for the Evaluation of Medicines (EMEA) and the Federal Food and Drug Administration (FDA). Guidance has been provided on the clinical investigation of medicinal products in the treatment of the indications under focus in this chapter, i.e. schizophrenia (CIMP, 1998), bipolar disorder (CIMP, 2005), depression (CDER, 1997; CIMP, 2002), and anxiety disorder (CDER, 1977; CIMP, 2005). Recommendations are provided on the use of placebo, efficacy criteria, methods to assess efficacy, choice of instruments, the study population, study design, strategy, safety, and special populations (i.e. children, adolescents, and elderly patients).

The debate continues on the use of placebo in clinical trials in psychiatry. The EMEA would argue on the one hand that such a design is required to define the "absolute" effects of a product; however, it raises an ethical issue if effective treatments are available to patients. That said, it would be unacceptable ethically to grant an approval in the absence of unambiguous evidence. The FDA guidance document indicates that the use of placebo in conditions such as depression and anxiety poses a problem in that the superiority of standard existing drugs over placebo is modest, thus rendering the administration of placebo to some patients in a study entirely justifiable. An explicit provision for removing patients from a study whose clinical condition worsens or fails to improve in a reasonable period of time is recommended. In schizophrenia, new products are being developed whereas the concept of the disorder and the diagnostic and efficacy criteria have changed; thus the efficacy of the older products may not be a useful indicator. Furthermore, the newer compounds may have a different effect on negative symptoms or extrapyramidal side effects, which may confound the efficacy analysis. The EMEA thus conclude that, in principle, placebo-controlled trials will be required to show efficacy, but discussion around alternative suitable designs should not be excluded.

Disorders should be classified according to the *Diagnostic and Statistical Manual* (American Psychiatric Association, 2000). In line with the EMEA guidance, a detailed history of the duration of disorder, severity, duration of the current episode, the number of episodes per time interval, and previous treatment outcome should be documented for all patients entering a trial. In addition baseline rating scores on instruments (e.g. PANSS, HAM-D, YMRS, etc.) should be defined in the protocol inclusion criteria.

Consideration is also given to licensing claims and the need for homogeneous populations, e.g.:

- If a claim on negative symptoms is to be made, specific trials should be conducted with predominant and persistent negative symptoms; stable patients for > 6 months, flat affect, and poverty of speech represent core negative symptoms, though the extent may differ between patients; major depression should be excluded; account for effects on EPS.

- If a claim is to be made for schizoaffective patients, then specific trials are required.
- Major depression may be further defined into mild, moderate, and severe and additional studies in severe patients may lead to additional claims. Typically trials address moderately ill patients as it is difficult to demonstrate an effect in mildly depressed patients.

Table 1 provides an overview of the key considerations provided by the EMEA and should be borne in mind when finalizing protocols to support claims in the various indications.

In light of the ethical issues raised, it is imperative that the impact of the study is limited by ensuring a minimum duration and continued possibility of withdrawing a patient in the event of deterioration. In the case of the latter, standard therapy should be given.

Recommendations are also provided for special populations and the requirements for specific studies. For example in elderly patients, data may be extrapolated from the total patient population (of all ages) or indeed a separate trial may be required if dealing with a compound with a new mode of action. Efficacy and safety in young adolescents are highly desirable in schizophrenia and bipolar disorder; however, in GAD the prevalence is low in adolescents and it does not seem to occur in children, hence rendering trial conduct very difficult although interest has increased over the past few years.

Recent literature has indicated that only 30% of schizophrenic patients are compliant in clinical trials, thus all steps should also be taken to improve compliance; e.g.:

- monitoring plasma levels
- counting tablets
- screening for use of illicit psychotropic substances.

All adverse events need to be recorded during the course of the study. In terms of long-term safety, the dossier must include data on a large and representative group of patients. In the case of depression, specific attention should be paid to the possibility of suicides and, where relevant, serotonergic syndrome. Furthermore, any information available on accidental overdose or deliberate self-poisoning should be provided. Special efforts should be made to assess adverse effects of the class of products.

When performing US trials, reference should also be made to the FDA guidelines for the clinical evaluation of antidepressant drugs and antianxiety drugs. There are no guidelines for the evaluation of antipsychotics at this time. The guidance documents from the FDA have many similarities with the EMEA guidance documents, although are structured differently and according to phases of development. Guidance is provided on general methodology, ethics, data collection, monitoring, and design issues per phase of development.

According to FDA guidance in antidepressants and anxiolytics, up to five double-blind trials in Phase III should compare the new compound with a placebo and a comparator in a similar pharmacological class. Long-term safety studies may be open-label or of a controlled parallel group design and may be as long as a year in duration.

Contrary to the EMEA guidance, whilst it is claimed that there is considerable interest in maintenance of effect trials, there is no recommendation that these studies should be conducted. Some of the problems associated with this type of design are related to the identification of patients likely to suffer from multiple recurrences and attrition owing to the duration of the trial.

Table 1.

Indication	Placebo use	Study considerations	Study design	Special groups	Endpoints
Schizophrenia	In principle placebo-controlled trials required but suitable alternative designs may be discussed with the competent authorities	In acute exacerbation, a double-blind phase of at least 6 weeks is generally considered adequate proof of efficacy	Treatment should be preceded by a washout that is sufficiently long to allow elimination of compounds	No specific trials required for geriatric patients or younger children, although efficacy and safety in young adolescents are highly desirable	PANSS
	For negative symptoms, there is no "gold standard" reference therapy, thus a placebo-controlled design is necessary. Inclusion of a comparator is recommended	Double-blind extension studies may be performed and should last 1 year.	Concomitant medications should be well documented		SANS
		Or a relapse prevention study may be conducted (duration of the acute phase needs to be longer than 6 weeks with an open-label stabilization phase).	Steps should be taken to minimize drop-outs		BPRS
		If a claim on negative symptoms is to be made, specific trials should be conducted with predominant and persistent negative symptoms; stable patients for > 6 months, flat affect, and poverty of speech represent core negative symptoms, though the extent may differ			Clinical Global Impression, item 2 of the CGI as a secondary endpoint

Depression	Three-arm trials including a placebo and an active control are recommended	between patients; major depression should be excluded; account for effects on EPS. If a claim is to be made for schizoaffective patients, then specific trials are required. Relapse prevention studies may be used to demonstrate that the effect is maintained, but is not a claim in itself	Limit duration of treatment	For elderly patients, the "optimal" design is a placebo-controlled response study. Data may, however, be extracted from a whole database	HAM-D (preferably 17-item)
		About 6 weeks should be sufficient treatment and anything longer justified			
		For licensing, maintenance of effect should be shown. A relapse prevention study is advisable with a duration of 8–12 weeks during the first period and randomization for up to 6 months	Fail-safe provision to allow withdrawal in the event of deterioration and provision of standard therapy	For children, trials should address children and adolescents	MADRS
		No specific guidance exists for treatment-resistant patients;	For relapse prevention, include specific measures to prevent complications		Item 2 of the CGI

Table 1. (cont.)

Indication	Placebo use	Study considerations	Study design	Special groups	Endpoints
		however, pivotal trials are recommended to include placebo and/or an acceptable comparator	of the disease, especially suicide		Rating scales should be specific for children and adolescents
			Consider close monitoring, and rescue medication.		
			For treatment-resistant patients, a prospective treatment duration is required and should be sufficiently long as non-compliance should not be the underlying cause of resistance		
Bipolar disorder	Three-arm trials including a placebo and an active control are recommended	Effect of a product in the acute phase and prevention of further episodes should be addressed.	For short-term trials to assess mania, preferably patients with only an episode should be included.	In adolescents, efficacy and safety evaluation is highly desirable.	Manic State Rating Scale for manic episodes
		Claims may be made for the following indications: (a) treatment of manic/depressive episodes and prevention of both or (b) a license for the treatment of manic episodes and prevention of manic/depressive episodes separately or	To demonstrate recurrence, it is recommended to include patients with a reasonably high recurrence rate. Patients should be free of manic/depressive symptoms for a sustained period of time		Young Mania Rating Scale for manic episodes

Indication	Study design	Long-term studies	Placebo / wash-out	Specific considerations	Rating scales / endpoints
	(c) a license for episodes of major depression in the framework of bipolar disorder		In bipolar depression, to make a monotherapy claim, patients must be off lithium or other mood stabilizers for a substantial period of time to avoid possible rebound phenomena		HAM-D, MADRS for switching from mania to depression
Generalized anxiety disorder	At least 8-week parallel, double-blind, randomized placebo controlled studies are necessary. Three-arm trials including a placebo and an active control are recommended	In addition to short-term trials (8 week treatment), relapse prevention studies are required. The open phase is at least 2 months and the randomization phase up to 12 months	A placebo run-in period to exclude placebo responders is useful A wash-out of current treatments is required	Efficacy and safety in elderly patients may be derived from the total database Defining a safe dose may be a concern, thus optimal to perform a placebo-controlled dose-response study A separate trial may also be required if the compound has a new mode of action	Hamilton anxiety rating scale (HAM-A) as a primary endpoint Using a structured interview may be useful (i.e. MINI) Secondary endpoints: – HAM-A psychic and somatic anxiety factor – Sheehan Disability scale – CGI

Upfront planning

Missing an NDA timeline is not an option. Evidence-based planning, effective implementation, and risk management are key to the successful delivery of a clinical plan. Key areas to assess from the outset are:

1. Protocol feasibility
2. Patient recruitment potential
3. Competitive environment
4. Country selection
5. Investigative site selection
6. Scenario planning
7. Risk management.

First and foremost, protocols must be in compliance with the above-mentioned FDA and EMEA guidance documents. Inclusion of a placebo arm will significantly influence the ability to conduct a trial. Whilst in accordance with regulators, ethical committees in certain countries may not accept such a protocol design (see Start-up section beginning on page 136). CNS trials with a placebo arm have typically been widely accepted in the USA, Eastern Europe, and Asia and to this end sponsors should give thought to including such regions when striving to meet rigid timelines. Countries typically rejecting pure placebo trials may, however, be open to considering "prevention of relapse studies" which allow for an open-label period of treatment for 2 months followed by a randomization to either the trial compound or a placebo. Inclusion of an open-label extension is clearly of benefit to the patients and welcomed by ethical committees. When selecting countries, it is advisable to investigate upfront on acceptability of trial design. It should be borne in mind that authorities may change their perspective and thus it is also recommended to have contingent countries identified from the outset.

The best feasibility study is often derived from the most recently completed trial. Whilst it is imperative to seek investigator and key opinion leader input when launching into new indications, it is widely recognized that investigator ability to predict recruitment potential is often variable. Over the past decade, thousands of clinical trials have been conducted in the CNS field with a particular focus on schizophrenia, bipolar disorder, generalized anxiety disorder, and major depressive disorder (clinicaltrials.gov). More recently, trials have focused also on schizoaffective disorder and bipolar depression. Where recruitment data are available, it is imperative that an analysis of past performance be conducted against similar inclusion/exclusion criteria. Clinical trial management systems typically permit access to site performance in terms of recruitment rates, screen failure rates, randomization rates, and patient retention. More sophisticated tools allow companies to drill down into specific searches linked to trial design, placebo arms, and concomitant medications. Finally, data on site performance related to separation data should be reviewed (see section below).

This alone, however, is insufficient as the competitive environment will also have a significant influence on the ability to conduct and complete a trial. The biggest risk of delay occurs when many sponsors are competing for the same patients in the same countries and in the same timeframe. Resources at the site level will also ultimately become a limiting factor.

The introduction of clinicaltrials.gov should not be ignored as it has ensured complete transparency with respect to competing trials, the latter having a significant impact on recruitment potential. A comprehensive assessment of ongoing trials should be conducted

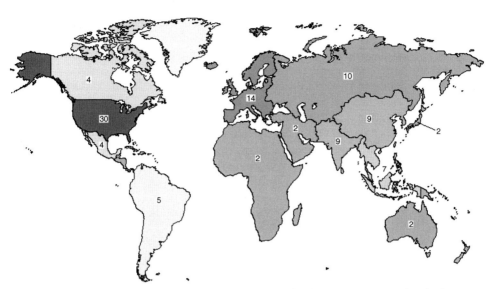

Figure 1. Clinical trial research activity in schizophrenia. Number of trials per region. Source: clinicaltrials.gov, Dec. 2009. See plate section for color version.

when selecting countries; for example, currently there are 41 industry-sponsored, interventional Phase II and III studies listed worldwide, with the highest competition for patients in North America and Europe (Figure 1). Patient participation in Asia has expanded over the past 2–3 years and it is increasingly becoming a region of choice for marketing as well as recruitment opportunities. Thus, when planning for a global program a more refined search may be conducted to assess on a country and site level where the competition lies.

In the absence of hard data, thought should be given to conducting a feasibility study via investigator sites and key opinion leaders. A combination of practicing physicians and key opinion leaders yields a balanced analysis of protocol feasibility and may often be complemented by focus groups regionally (i.e. practicing physicians are invited to contribute to roundtable discussions on key protocol issues). This also ensures engagement at the site level at an early stage in the process. A questionnaire is designed to capture information on the protocol inclusion criteria, availability of patients, patient and caregiver interest, schedule of visits, investigator interest, concomitant medication, ethical considerations, experience with scales (e.g. the PANSS, SANS, CGI etc.), enrollment rates, logistics (e.g. MRIs, infusions, ECGs, clinical trial supply storage), personnel requirements, and grants. Availability of translated scales should also be assessed during the feasibility phase. In the absence of translations, time should be allowed to complete this step. An analysis of the feedback should in turn be used to ensure that the protocol is feasible and is amended as appropriate and that the timelines are attainable.

With continued advances in technology, feasibility studies are beginning to incorporate patient feedback in addition to investigator feedback. Reaching out to patients permits an analysis of patient interest in clinical research and also raises awareness of potential benefits to patients. An example of such technology is that of iguard.org, a drug safety monitoring service with access to patients diagnosed with schizophrenia. iguard.org will contact patients meeting the target profile and ask for their feedback via an online survey. Patients will give feedback on aspects of their condition, level of engagement in a trial, and materials developed to drive patient recruitment (messaging, branding campaigns, etc.).

Phase I trials in healthy volunteers are generally conducted in a minimum number of sites. Phase II trials and even more so Phase III programs require far more extensive planning and access to patients. Phase III CNS trials typically require inclusion of up to 4000 patients. With the increasing pressure to develop and launch, companies are required to consider global clinical trials. Country selection for Phase III programs is often based on a balance between the need for key marketing countries (e.g. USA, western Europe, and more recently China), recruitment potential (USA, eastern Europe, and Asia generally have the highest potential), prevalence of the indication and acceptability of the trial design and timelines (USA being the fastest to start up).

Study implementation
The start-up phase
In order to proceed with site initiations in countries, the following steps need to be undertaken:
- submission and approval from regulatory bodies
- submission and approval from ethical committees/IRBs
- clinical trial agreements and grants to be signed with investigators and/or hospitals/research institutions
- clinical trial logistics to be implemented (i.e. clinical trial supplies, IVRS, laboratory supplies, ECGs, etc.)
- training of site personnel (investigator meetings).

Approval requirements as well as the process vary from country to country but typically the following components constitute a submission package to regulatory authorities:
- Protocol and summary translated into local language
- Patient Information Leaflet and Consent Form
- Investigator's Brochure
- Insurance Certificate
- Certificate of Analysis
- Delegation letter
- Financial declaration
- Import license
- CVs of investigators
- Investigator grants
- For the USA, FDA 1571, 1572
- Drug applications include blank and executed batch manufacturing and packaging records
- Debarment statements; DMF authorization letters among many documents as part of the original (NDA, ANDA) or CTD application.

Timelines for approval are also country-specific and depend on whether submission to the regulatory bodies may be conducted in parallel or must be sequential (Table 2).

Table 2. Country process for regulatory and ethical submissions

Process	Country
Submissions to regulatory bodies and ethical committees in parallel	Argentina, Austria, Belgium, Bulgaria, Canada, Cyprus, Czech Rep., Denmark, Estonia, Finland, France, Germany, Hongkong, Hungary, Iceland, India, Ireland, Italy, Korea, Kuwait, Latvia, Lithuania, Malaysia, Malta, Netherlands, Norway, Paraguay, Peru, Philippines, Poland, Portugal, Romania, Russia, Rep. South Africa, Singapore, Slovakia, Sweden, Taiwan, Turkey, Ukraine, United Kingdom, United States, Venezuela
Sequential	Australia, Bosnia, Hercegovina, Brazil, China, Costa Rica, Croatia, Ecuador, Egypt, Greece, Guatemala, Honduras, Israel, Japan, Jordan, Lebanon, Mexico, Morocco, Panama, Saudi Arabia, Serbia, Slovenia, Spain, Switzerland, Thailand, United Arab Emirates, Uzbekistan, Vietnam
Partially sequential (at least one EC approval required prior to reg submission)	Chile, Colombia, Indonesia

Ensuring an efficient approval process requires careful planning. In general, regulatory and ethical bodies have fixed meeting dates to review submissions and thus should be anticipated. Questions from authorities should be anticipated and, where feasible, supporting documentation provided upfront (e.g. justificiation of a placebo arm). It cannot be assumed that approvals will be obtained first time round and indeed regulatory bodies may change their perspective on certain trial designs. Therefore it is advisable to build this assumption into the timeline scenario and furthermore to apply for approval in additional contingent countries upfront.

Time to approval varies significantly from country to country, the shortest being in the USA in 3 months if a central IRB is used. All other countries in Europe, Latin America, and Asia take approximately 4–9 months for full approval and this should be factored into the overall study timelines.

During this timeframe, it is advisable to ensure that clinical trial agreements and grants are in place at the site level. Sufficient time should be allowed to ensure legal review and agreement with hospital administration as appropriate. Investigator grants are fixed as a function of the labor involved to conduct patient visits (estimated according to number and duration of visits). Depending on the protocol, agreements may also need to be implemented with radiologists, ophthalmologists, or referring physicians. Travel costs should also be borne in mind for patients and caregivers if reimbursement is stipulated according to local legislation.

Both finalization of the protocol and the provision of clinical trial supplies is often rate-limiting in the start-up phase and companies should ensure that all manufacturing and packaging are planned well in advance. As for protocols, in the event of amendments, re-submissions may occur and may cause the clock to tick from day 1 again, depending on the country.

Table 3. Countries wherein a placebo design has been accepted in the respective indications based on the sample of studies analyzed (see Appendix 1)

Indication	Countries accepting placebo
Schizophrenia	Colombia, Costa Rica, France*, India, Indonesia, Lithuania, Japan, Malaysia, Mexico, Philippines, Russia, Romania, Taiwan, Slovakia*, South Africa, South Korea, Ukraine, USA
Bipolar disorder	Argentina (bipolar depression), Colombia, Costa Rica, Czech Republic (bipolar depression), France (bipolar depression), India, Indonesia, Lithuania, Japan, Malaysia, Mexico, Philippines, Russia, Romania, Taiwan, Serbia (bipolar depression), South Africa, South Korea, Ukraine, USA
Major depressive disorder	Argentina, Bulgaria*, Canada, Colombia, Denmark, Finland, France, Germany, India, Indonesia, Latvia, Lithuania, Japan, Malaysia, Mexico, Philippines, Poland*, Russia, Romania, Taiwan, South Africa, Serbia, South Korea, Slovakia, Spain*, Sweden, Turkey, Ukraine, UK*, USA
Generalized anxiety disorder	Argentina, Bulgaria, Canada, Chile, Colombia, Denmark, Finland, France, Germany, India, Indonesia, Lithuania, Japan, Malaysia, Mexico, Philippines, Poland*, Russia, Romania, Taiwan, South Africa, South Korea, Sweden, Spain*, Turkey, Ukraine, UK*, USA

* Schizophrenia: France: proven acceptance in 2007, strongly depends on design; Slovakia: proven acceptance in acute schizophrenia 10% probability for placebo, so depends on design.
MDD/GAD: Bulgaria: proven acceptance but climate changing, depends on design; Poland: climate is changing; until 2008 there has been a ban on placebo studies in psychiatry mainly due to suicide risk, nowadays acceptance depends on the design and minimizing the risks for the patients; hospitals can accept placebo design if patients can be hospitalized throughout the study; Spain and UK: have both acceptance and rejections so strongly depends on the design and minimizing risk.

Recruitment timelines and scenario planning

Recruitment periods are often determined working in reverse from a target NDA timeline. The recruitment timeframe is the time remaining after allowing for site start-up and removing time for the database lock, statistical analysis, provision of the final clinical report, and preparation of the filing. The number of sites required to meet the timeframe is established based on previous data or feasibility data.

Companies are investing more and more in sophisticated, algorithm-based modeling tools that incorporate real data to ensure precise planning. At a minimum, data on the following variables should be provided:

- number of months for ethical and regulatory approval in total
- screen failure rate per indication
- randomization rate per indication.

Table 4 provides an overview of average recruitment rates per site per country in key indications, based on the sample of studies provided in Appendix 1.

Assumptions should also be built in to allow for:

- the total number of sites (a statistical approach should be adopted to provide guidance on the maximum number of sites permissible)
- a staggered site initiation process (not all approvals will be provided at the same time and not all sites will be available for initiation simultaneously)

Table 4. Description of patient recruitment per indication

Indication	No. of studies	No. of unique sites	Total patients enrolled	Average recruitment rate per site per month
Schizophrenia	67	1417	25 261	1.1
Anxiety	25	614	9689	1.4
Bipolar disorder	17	312	5863	1.1
Major depressive disorder	14	381	12 510	1.2

Data have been extracted from the case study ($n = 123$ studies) and provide an overview of the number of studies, number of unique sites, total number of patients recruited, and the calculated average recruitment rate per site per month.

- target date for first patient to be accrued
- target date for last patient to be accrued
- seasonal fluctuations will have a significant impact on recruitment and should also be accommodated for (e.g. winter in RSA, Australia, July and August holidays in Europe, etc.)
- central versus local IRBs, as the latter take significantly longer to obtain approval.

Scenarios may in turn be generated as a function of the first patient in timeline and last patient in timeline. Depending on the overall recruitment timeline, patient forecasts may be projected on a weekly or monthly basis and thus monitored on an ongoing basis (example provided in Figure 3). Solutions to any delays from the original plan may thus be provided promptly.

The general pitfalls in timeline planning are related to:

- slower than planned-for approvals
- unexpected rejections from regulatory or ethical committees
- unexpected re-submissions
- lower than anticipated recruitment rates
- higher than anticipated screen failure rates
- non-recruiting sites.

Scenarios should be run for all of the above eventualities, and contingency plans provided upfront.

On average, based on the case study provided, up to 15% of sites do not recruit patients into trials and thus such a contingency should be built in upfront. Adding new sites during the course of the recruitment period may take at least 3 months to be activated. Given this, it is also advisable to plan for additional sites from the outset. From a management perspective, it is imperative to agree on timelines upfront and the timepoint at which additional intervention is required to ensure that timelines are still maintained.

Site selection

Site selection in any given clinical trial requires an evaluation of the following:

- investigator and co-investigator credentials, reputation, and research experience
- adequate staff and resources

- availability of appropriate facilities and equipment
- IRB services and turn-around time
- budget development and contract negotiations.

More specifically in trials in psychiatry, Kobak *et al.* (2004) depict the following skills as being necessary to participate in a clinical trial:

- conceptual understanding of the disorder of interest
- clinical experience with the population under study
- generic interviewing skills
- expertise in symptom rating scale administration
- understanding of the research milieu
- scale-specific expertise.

As mentioned above, the increasing challenge in conducting studies in psychiatric indications is the decreased signal detection that is observed in clinical trials. Whilst this used to be a problem for studies in major depressive disorders, in recent years several schizophrenia studies have also failed due to, amongst other factors, a high placebo response. This problem seems to be more prominent in the USA than in other countries; however, the issue seems to be spreading. Whilst there is no simple solution to this issue, in addition to the above criteria, companies are focusing more and more on analyzing site outcome in multinational trials and some of the larger CNS specialized clinical research organizations are building databases with such data, as they have a large sample size. Where sites have participated in previous trials in psychiatry it is useful to review whether they have provided conclusive data. Investigators are rarely provided with data on how they performed and indeed welcome such feedback. If a trial is conclusive, it is rare that the sponsor would return to discuss data from a site that may not have detected a signal. Whilst there is no guarantee, selecting sites which have experience in signal detection can only help to reduce risks of failure.

In a recent study by Merlo-Pich and Gomeni in 2008, the performance of each site was analyzed to provide criteria to discriminate between informative and non-informative centers using the signal detection approach. When reviewing a sample of nine multinational clinical trials in depression, they demonstrated that only 60% of sites were informative or indeed able to detect clinically relevant signals of efficacy. It was concluded that this type of methodology could be useful in future studies, provided the number of patients per site was sufficient (i.e. a minimum of four patients).

In addition, limiting the number of sites allows companies to choose the most experienced sites and at the same time reduce inter-rater variability. This, however, is not always an easy decision to make as companies are often so pressed to meet timelines and hence risk sacrificing quality.

Thus when selecting key investigative sites to participate in trials in psychiatry, in addition to reviewing their qualifications, GCP training, facilities, patient population etc., it is critical to understand how they have performed in signal detection in previous trials.

Investigator training

Efficacy in psychiatry trials is assessed by means of rating scales. Both the FDA (1998) and EMEA (1998) guidelines clearly make reference to the need to address factors such as content validity, inter- and intra-rater reliability, and responsiveness for detecting changes in the severity of disease when instruments are selected for primary efficacy assessments.

Complementary to this, the EMEA guidance indicates that:

- investigators should be properly trained in evaluating the patient
- in multi-center/multi-investigator studies inter-rater reliability scores (kappa) should be documented for each investigator in advance and during the study both with regard to the diagnosis and to rating scales used for efficacy and/or safety, where relevant
- the PANSS and SANSS should be used only if inter-rater reliability studies are performed in advance and during the studies and if the inter-rater reliability scores for the negative symptoms are satisfactory.

Kobak *et al.* (2005) argue that this alone is not sufficient, but that interviewing skills have a profound effect on signal detection. In the study conducted, paroxetine failed to separate from placebo overall; however, subjects whose interviews were rated good to excellent separate paroxetine from placebo.

The case for standardizing the use of clinical rated outcome measures to improve outcome is not new (Butler, 2009), but at a minimum sponsors need to invest in training programs to ensure investigators are trained on rating scales and certified, that kappa values are documented, and that interviewing skills are appropriate to pick up on signal detection.

Managing recruitment

Having finalized the trial design, selected countries, gained approvals, and initiated investigative sites, managing recruitment at the site level is a central component of study conduct. As previously mentioned, only 70% of studies meet the original study timelines and the costs of such delays are far from negligible. Thus, the process of finding, screening, enrolling, and retaining large numbers of clinical trial patients simultaneously at multiple research sites in multiple countries is a challenge for even the largest pharmaceutical sponsors and clinical research organizations. Enrollment of patients known to sites generally represents the early accrual at the site level; however, this pool is often exhausted prematurely and may not also be counted on to meet rigid timelines. Waiting for patients to walk in the door is a high risk and onerous option. It is advisable to work with specialists in the field of patient recruitment and retention who can design a customized campaign for the study. It is important to emphasize that one size does not fit all and a tailored approach is required per indication and per country and even per site. Finding severely depressed treatment-resistant patients or schizophrenic patients with prominent negative symptoms is clearly a challenge as these patients are more likely to be at home and unwilling to seek help or social interactions compared to the mildly depressed or patients with acute episodes of schizophrenia.

Thus at the outset of a study or program, thought should be given to the following:

- creation and production of study specific recruitment materials
- creation and placement of public relations campaigns
- design and management of direct mail campaigns
- management of a centralized call center for pre-screening potential patients, which, in turn, would require the following:
  - development of standardized pre-screening script(s)
  - daily referrals to study sites
  - scheduling of screening visits (first visit) to sites as desired by site/sponsor

- site follow-up on referrals and continuous site support during campaign
- a full complement of reports for call activity, media success, and referrals made
- coordination of IRB/EC approvals for all recruitment and retention materials
- coordination of translation of materials into other languages.

It is key that investigators and study monitors allow sufficient time to develop a recruitment plan at the site level and that it is reviewed on an ongoing basis during the accrual period.

Introducing a competitive approach to patient recruitment, in addition to the closure of non-performing sites, can be helpful in ensuring site motivation. Active management of sites will also ensure that as the studies approach recruitment targets, sites will either be "capped" or informed of revised patient targets to ensure that the study does not over-recruit, potentially eroding the power of the study.

Eligible patients

Diagnosis being complex and co-morbidities frequent in psychiatry (e.g. GAD, with a lifetime co-morbidity among 90.4% of the people who had a history of GAD), trial management methodology should focus on patient eligibility. Investigators and site co-ordination staff should be trained on the diagnostic tools and protocol-specific inclusion and exclusion criteria. Where patient eligibility is considered to be a high risk in relation to trial outcome, thought should be given to proactively reviewing patients being entered into the trial. Such a review may be conducted via the provision of pre-screening logs and discussed with medical monitors devoted to the study trial. The following information should be collated at a minimum to allow a monitor to review patient eligibility and provide approval to enter the trial:

- date of diagnosis
- description of symptoms
- description of associated psychiatric symptoms
- description of current psychosocial situations
- whether symptoms have been stable, and if so for how long
- list current and past treatments and doses taken
- date of hospitalization and reason for hospitalization
- describe adverse events experienced by the patient, including EPS
- whether the patient has participated in previous trials.

Technology should allow a speedy review of the patient inclusion at the site level as described in the process below. Once a patient has been pre-identified, the investigator enters criteria into an electronic data capture system. An alert is in turn sent to a medical monitor, who may approve or disapprove entrance into the trial. If the patient's screening visit is approved, an immediate alert is sent to the investigator to ensure that no time is lost when treating patients.

It is also key to ensure that steps are taken to avoid enrolling the same patient in multiple trials (commonly known as "the professional patient"). Clearly the question should be asked of the patient upfront, but thought should also be given to building in data management checks on the demographic data both within studies and across programs.

Monitoring quality

Managing quality during the course of a clinical trial may only be achieved via robust clinical, data management, and project plans.

Monitors typically visit investigative sites on a monthly basis (or more if recruitment is higher than expected, or less if the study is an open-label extension with wider patient visit intervals) to verify:

- compliance with the protocol
- compliance with ICH/GCP guidance
- that the process of obtaining informed consent has been respected
- review of medical records against the protocol to ensure patient eligibility
- reporting of laboratory data, adverse events, serious adverse events, and concomitant medication
- drug accountability and compliance.

Data are collected via case report forms and the data management plan outlines data flow and validation checks to be conducted on the data. Monitors are obliged to perform the following activities:

- review the data collected against medical records or source documentation at the investigative site level and
- address data inconsistencies via queries issued resulting from validation checks as consensus must be reached with the investigators.

Monitoring plans are written to define the extent of data verification and typically characterize data as being critical or non-critical. In the case of the former, 100% data verification is required by the monitor, whereas for non-critical data 25% data verification may be acceptable. More and more companies are also using sampling techniques to validate data (Williams, 2006).

Depending on the nature of the trial and compound under development, unblinded review of efficacy and safety parameters may be required on an ongoing basis. To ensure that the validity of the trial is respected, data monitoring committees (DMC) or data safety monitoring boards (DSMB) may be established independently and meet on a pre-determined frequency. Guidelines are established upfront to define the variables to be reviewed and the stopping guidelines.

Measuring success

It is well recognized that monitoring of key performance indicators (KPIs) drives performance and study improvement and permits identification of issues across studies or programs on an ongoing basis. Whilst there is no consensus on key performance indicators for a given trial, a selection of the following KPIs should be considered:

From a timeline perspective, the following metrics are generally reviewed:

- time from final protocol to first site initiated
- time to first patient in
- time to 50% of patients recruited
- time to last patient in
- time from last patient last visit to database lock

- time to high-level results
- time to the clinical study report.

From a patient perspective:
- number of eligible patients
- number of days hospitalization
- number of relapses
- number of deviations from the protocol.

From a data quality perspective:
- number of queries per site
- number or percentage of database errors.

From the site level:
- number of non-recruiting sites.

Clinical trial management systems allow companies to have online access to these parameters and to issue dashboards for management review.

Summary and conclusion

When managing clinical trials in psychiatry, generation of the right strategy is critical to successful trial implementation. Where possible, such a strategy should be evidence-based. Consideration should be given to trial design (phase, placebo arm, chronic versus acute settings, patient visits, inpatient settings etc.), regulatory and ethical acceptance of the trial, patient recruitment rates, investigator performance, competing trials, availability of translated scales, and interest in the trial.

Missing an NDA timeline is not an option so scenario planning should be conducted upfront and where possible be data-driven (i.e. based on recruitment metrics, time to regulatory and ethical approval, competing trials, central versus local IRBs, seasonal variations etc.). Such a modeling exercise permits the identification of required contingencies upfront and provides assurance in the event of non-recruiting sites and non-approval by regulatory or ethical bodies. When dealing with challenging patient settings (e.g. severely depressed patients, treatment-resistant patients), a tailored recruitment strategy should be considered and may require advertising campaigns.

Diagnosis being complex and co-morbidities frequent in psychiatry, trial management methodology should focus on patient eligibility. Investigators and site coordination staff should be trained on the diagnostic tools and protocol-specific inclusion and exclusion criteria. Where patient eligibility is considered to be high risk in relation to trial outcome, thought should be given to proactively reviewing patients being entered into the trial. Such a review may be conducted via the provision of pre-screening logs and discussed with medical monitors devoted to the study trial. Trial monitors should also be trained to ensure that patient eligibility and severity is monitored during the course of the trial.

Trial management in psychiatry is further complicated by the fact that there are no hard endpoints and thus efficacy is based on subjective measurements via validated rating scales. Whilst guidance from a regulatory standpoint is vague, investigators must be trained on the

Global Psychiatry Performance

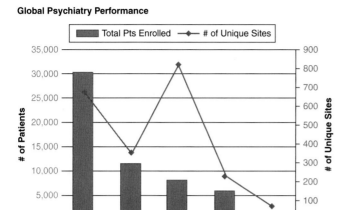

Figure 2. Total number of patients and unique recruiting sites. Data have been collected from trials conducted in schizophrenia ($n = 67$), bipolar disorder ($n = 17$), major depressive disorder ($n = 14$), and generalized anxiety disorder ($n = 25$) during the period 1997 to 2008. The total number of patients recruited per region and the total number of unique sites contributing is depicted over the period 1997–2008. The number of studies is illustrated beside each region, e.g. CEE 57 studies.

relevant scales in advance of any trial. Training has evolved over the past decade and focuses not only on inter-rater reliability but also on administering patient interviews.

In summary, with the increasing pressure on companies to reduce time to market coupled with the risk of failed outcomes, CNS trial management should focus on outcome data (signal detection), evidence-based planning, patient eligibility, and dealing with subjective endpoints.

Acknowledgements

The author extends sincere thanks to Cathy Vanbelle, Director of CNS Therapeutics at Quintiles, who conducted the analysis and provided the graphs for the case study.

Appendix 1

Figure 2 illustrates the total number of patients recruited, the total number of investigational sites involved, and the number of studies per indication. Sites in North America followed by central and eastern Europe (CEE) have contributed most to clinical research in psychiatry during the period 1997–2008 and sites in Asia and Latin America (AAA) are becoming more and more involved. Whilst the number of potential sites is high in western Europe (WE), patient accrual has often been impacted by trial design and competition for patients.

The regional contribution per indication is significantly different. Figure 3 provides an overview of the regional contribution to patient recruitment per indication. North America has dominated the field of MDD with a contribution of 83% of all patients whereas AAA and CEE made minor contributions of 3 and 4% respectively and western Europe 10%. The contribution of WE increased significantly in the field of anxiety disorders (40%) with NA contributing almost equally. CEE, however, has largely contributed to developments in schizophrenia and bipolar depression and mania. Similarly, the AAA region made a major contribution particularly in bipolar disorders (32%).

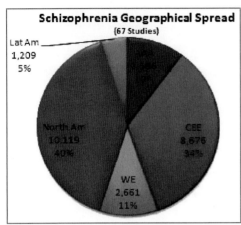

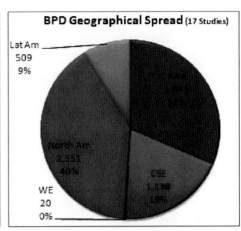

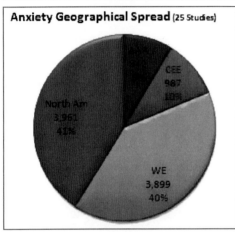

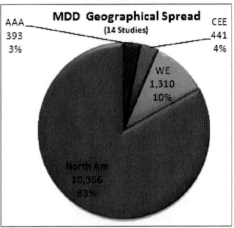

Figure 3. Patients recruited per indication per region. See plate section for color version.

References

Andrews, G. (2001). Placebo response in depression: bane of research, boon to therapy. *Brit J Psychiat*, 178, 192–4.

Antonuccio, D., Burns, D., and Danton, W. G. (2002). Antidepressants: a triumph of marketing over science. Commentary on The Emperor's New Drugs: an analysis of antidepressant medication data submitted to the U.S. Food and Drug Administration. *Prevention Treatment*, 5 (25), 1–21.

Brown, W. (1995). The placebo response in depression: a modest proposal. *Harvard Mental Health Letter*, 12, 6.

Butler, A. (2009). Seeking guidance on rater reliability. *Appl Clin Trials*, 18, 1.

Center for Drug Evaluation and Research, Guidance for Industry (Feb 1977). Guidelines for the clinical evaluation of Antianxiety Drugs.

Center for Drug Evaluation and Research, Guidance for Industry (Feb 1997). Guidelines for the clinical evaluation of Antidepressant Drugs.

Clinical Investigation of Medicinal Products in the Treatment of Schizophrenia (Aug 1998) CPMP/EWP/559/95.

Clinical Investigation of Medicinal Products for the treatment and prevention of Bipolar Disorder (Oct 2001) CPMP/EWP/567/98.

Clinical Investigation of Medicinal Products indicated for Generalised Anxiety Disorder (Jul 2005). CPMP/EWP/4284/02.

Clinical Investigation of Medicinal Products in the Treatment of Depression (Oct 2002). CPMP/EWP/518/97 Rev. 1.

Cutting Edge Information (Oct 2004) *NewsRx. com & NewsRx.net.*

Diagnostic and Statistical Manual of Mental Disorders DSM-IV-TR (2000). American Psychiatric Association, 4th edition.

FDA Center for Drug Evaluation and Research, Guidance for Industry (1998). E9 Statistical Principles for Clinical Trials, ICH ratified.

Forest Laboratories, Safety Update, Regulatory Status Update (1998) World Literature Update [Correspondence]. US Food and Drug Administration, 1–108.

ICH (September 1998) E9 Statistical Principles for Clinical Trials. CPMP/ICH/363/96.

Ker, A., Stadler, J., and Viljoen, M. (2000). The role of placebo and the placebo response in clinical research. *Geneeskunde. Med J*, 42, 8.

Kirby, L., Borwege, S., Christensen, J., Weber, C., and McCarthy, C. (2005) *Appl Clin Trials.*

Kirsch, I., Moore, T. J., Scoboria, A., and Nicholls, S. S. (2002). The Emperor's New Drugs: an analysis of antidepressant medication data submitted to the US Food and Drug Administration. *Prevention Treatment*, 5 (23).

Kobak, K. A., Engelhardt, N., Williams, J. B., and Lipsitz, J. D. (2004). Rater training in multicenter clinical trials: issues and recommendations. *J Clin Psychopharmacol*, 24, 113–17.

Kobak, K. A., Feiger, A. D., and Lipsitz, J. D. (2005). Interview quality and signal detection in clinical trials. *Am J Psychiat*, 162, 628.

Lane, R. (1999). Placebo response to antidepressants. *Ger J Psychiatr*, 2 (3), 1–11.

Laughren, T. P. (1998). Recommendation for approval action for Celexa (citalopram) for the treatment of depression [Memorandum]. US Food and Drug Administration, 1–5.

Lipton, L. (2000). Placebo response can confound drug trials. *Psychiatric News*. July.

Merlo-Pich, E. and Gomeni, R. (2008). Model-based approach and signal detection theory to evaluate the performance of recruitment centers in clinical trials with antidepressant drugs. *Clin Pharmacol Therapeut*, 84(3), 378–84.

Oosterbaan, D. B., van Balkom, A. J., Spinhoven, P., and Van Dyck, R. (2001). The placebo response in social phobia. *J Psychopharmacol*, 15 (3), 199–203.

Williams, G. W. (2006). The other side of clinical trial monitoring; assuring data quality and procedural adherence. *Clin Trials*, 3, 530–7.

Clinical trials management at the site level

Joseph Kwentus

Introduction and history

Earlier chapters have defined the steps in preclinical drug development and phases of clinical trial testing. This chapter explains common practices and customs at the CNS drug trial site, a complex ingredient in the recipe for new medicines.

The CNS research site

Sponsors perform clinical trials for many reasons. Companies plan trials for winning approval for new drugs or for proving novel uses for present ones. Further, sponsors run trials to clarify dosing, learn about long-term safety, or position products in the marketplace. And all of these studies must follow complex rules which vary from country to country.

Each year, trials are more complex and difficult. In this decade, the number of procedures per clinical trial increased by 49% and effort needed to carry out procedures grew by 54%. Central nervous trials saw rapid growth in the total number of procedures and the burden to perform them. Time-consuming procedures make it more difficult for subjects to finish individual sessions and discourage them from completing the study (Getz et al., 2008). Detailed inclusion and exclusion lists lessen the number of available volunteers, and sites have more difficulty finding and recruiting subjects. Thus, trial sites must be flexible, identify the right subjects, and measure the core variables correctly.

The organization diagram of most trial sites is simple. The critical ingredients are the principal investigator and the clinical coordinators. Community outreach staff, business support workers, and rating specialists round out the team. To carry out some medical procedures, the investigator needs to call on consultants in non-CNS areas. Radiology, ophthalmology, endocrinology, or dermatology may play supporting roles in some studies. Some sites perform many different kinds of trials; others specialize in definite disorders, such as depression or schizophrenia. Sites with focused expertise may dedicate themselves only to performing work in specific areas, such as abuse liability, therapeutic classrooms, imaging, or sleep. Investigators conduct CNS clinical trials in diverse local settings, various size businesses, and different national cultures. Success depends on the talents of people with various backgrounds, training, and experience. Doctors prescribe for patients who live in many different environments; therefore, research settings parallel the clinic setting where patients are likely to take the medicines.

Essential CNS Drug Development, ed. A. Kalali, Sheldon Preskorn, J. Kwentus, and Stephen M. Stahl.
Published by Cambridge University Press. © Cambridge University Press 2012.

Because sites do trials in diverse settings, the sponsor must do everything possible to help sites be consistent and reliable. The drug developer's true mission is to find sites that can do specific studies well. Every site must be able to enroll qualified subjects and assess core scales faithfully. To this end, most studies have a communication plan that includes meetings, rater training, newsletters, and contact with sponsor staff. Sponsors have to guarantee sites follow FDA rules and guidelines, so companies sometimes talk to sites more about compliance than data. Sites and sponsors rarely discuss budgets after startup, but budgets are also important in completing trials. Since most sites are small businesses, running with limited capital, they must analyze hidden costs and know how they are going to pay for them. However, even in institutions with deep pockets, like universities or multispecialty clinics, the study must come in within budget. Sites analyze costs ahead of time and should know how to run the study within the budget. Promoting the study, long visits, and transport can cause costs that may be difficult to predict.

Clinical trials can be worthwhile for investigators. In academic settings, young doctors often have their first research experience carrying out a role in a trial. In private practice, industry-funded trials allow doctors to be on the front line of medicine, without being part of a full-time university faculty. The investigator is the real-world link between the patient and the drug developer. Therefore, recruiting well-qualified investigators is a major goal of industry. The principal investigator ought to be a hard-working individual who is steadfast, honest, and careful. This role calls for someone who is a skilled supervisor and has mastery of the related medical specialty. Since the ability to exchange ideas skillfully is the key to success, the researcher must display respect, patience, tact, and openness. Although a scientific background is critical to the mission, the researcher must show concern and empathy for the participant's anguish. To reassure patients about taking part in a study, the investigator displays respect for their attitudes and appreciation of their difficulty. Investigators must be self-aware, displaying restraint when discussing either the product or project. They must remain neutral by continually teaching the staff about the illness and the goals of the study. This calls for strong enduring associations with employees, referrers, and participants.

Investigators are responsible for everything that happens in a study, but coordinators make the study happen. The coordinator gets the project on track and ensures the staff, consultants, and third-party services work together. Coordinators clarify what everyone needs to do and when he or she needs to do it. Coordinators work as project managers during study startup and as line managers when the study is running. As both investigator and coordinator share successes or failures, communication between the two must be clear. The coordinator must immediately express project-related needs to the investigator. The investigator directs the study and makes sure the people, tools, and supplies to do the study are accessible. Time management is the most important skill the coordinator can bring to the table. The coordinator foresees obstacles, plans solutions, and makes sure that staff act reliably. Every journey needs a map. The site policy and procedure manual is the site's road map for completing projects. This manual unites the site staff with common principles that apply to all projects. Effective coordinators use this manual as a living document to complete studies and work with the investigator to revise it when necessary. The coordinator helps staff see the goal and engages in a win-win with investigator, sponsor, and CRO. Veteran coordinators, seasoned in CNS research, must spend years mentoring junior employees for them to become qualified.

Training is the key to site success. FDA demands the investigator assign trial roles and train the staff. Well-trained staff teach research subjects how to give unbiased reports of their symptoms and carry out the research. They remind participants that research is different from going to the doctor to get treatment. A well-done study helps the subjects pay more attention to symptoms and improves their awareness of their disease. Once the trial is over, a research participant will have learned skills that help them collaborate in medical care.

The arrangement between the sites and the sponsor

To get the privilege to test a candidate drug, a research site presents itself to a suitable sponsor. To start, the site goes to the sponsor's website and provides information about its interests and abilities. Sites need to learn when new projects are starting. Sites then need to get in touch with key decision-makers before they select who will do the study. Sites must have well-timed updates about new products and emerging indications. Databases such as clinical trials.gov or CenterWatch give basic information. However, the most useful leads come from personal associations. Going to scientific meetings provides up-to-date technical news and offers the possibility for chance meetings with thought leaders and decision-makers. Professional business developers help sites find studies, but are expensive. Backing by a well-respected investigator can be helpful for newer research sites trying to prove themselves. A veteran site checks its competence by frequent self-audits. Sites must shine in business behavior, compliance, presentation, and scientific conduct. Repeat business from satisfied sponsors is not only the benchmark of success, but research sites perform best when they pick up a drug early and stay with it throughout the product life cycle.

Recruitment

Recruitment is clearly central to the success of any trial. The first published template of a recruitment plan occurred in 1992 (Spilker and Cramer, 1992). The plan recognized that the number of people likely to enter is usually much less than estimates. Often, a suitable group seems available, but the site and sponsor fail to realize how much eligibility rules shrink the numbers of valid patients. Successful sites embrace plans that recognize that only a fraction of people who inquire about the trial will screen. Of those who screen, a smaller number will randomize and still fewer complete the study.

Researchers use creative marketing methods to find volunteers to take part in studies. Newer tools for finding subjects include email lists, direct mail, data banks, digital media, and social media, among others. Subjects take part in studies freely, but the final decision usually rests on a few details that motivate them to commit. Some hope the study will bring them a cure, others that it will advance therapies for future patients. Most participants take part in a study only when they identify its personal relevance. When subjects understand what the study expects to achieve, they can put it in an individual context. Staff should have a clear understanding of the subject's reason for getting involved. When staff show empathy and respect, participants increase trust. When investigators encourage staff to be obliging and flexible, patients become open to the possibilities. Staff nurture patients to trust by listening. Participants, their families, and their caregivers all have unique points of view. When the staff understand these viewpoints, they can describe the study and answer questions clearly. Staff should encourage participants to look at the disadvantages of the study as well as benefits before agreeing to enter. Once certain the subject knows what the study has to offer, the staff must decrease barriers that hinder involvement. The usual barriers involve time, travel, and trouble.

The unique character of the site controls the access to recruitment. Major medical centers rely heavily on their databases. At the other extreme, some dedicated research sites rely on media campaigns. However, the most successful sites exploit various methods that build on one another. Whether the site relies on an internal data bank, a community outreach program, or advertising, foresight is necessary. The plan begins when the site puts the last touches on the feasibility survey. If the sponsor sets up the feasibility review poorly, the site should answer with its own enrollment plan, addressing major issues. Sites may either share plans with the sponsor, or file them for use when the study launches. For instance, enquiries about site databases are relevant when the disorder under scrutiny is stable schizophrenia. However, if the study is about acute episodes, links the site has with emergency rooms and crisis teams apply more directly. In this case, the investigator can let the sponsor know the number in the database, but also make the sponsor aware of dealings with emergency rooms and crisis teams. A marketing plan that clarifies key issues should be available before startup.

Marketing plans rarely mention word of mouth as a referral tool. However, local reputation is one important reason that a patient will decide to call a research practice. Participants, former patients, and families will exchange opinions. These conversations occur in waiting rooms, in the lunchroom, at the hospital, and at work. When research produces an unfavorable result, it is critical to be honest and remind subjects about the goals of research. Participants recognize that research efforts contribute to treatments in the future and that sometimes even existing treatments have poor results. It is more important that the research staff treat subjects with respect. Participants who feel well treated pass along their experiences in favorable terms. When word gets out, it creates sensible, clear expectations in the community. In an age of social media, information spreads at light speed and a good name makes all the difference.

The research message is the medium. To gain a great name, a research site must be exactly as it appears. The investigator must create interest in studies, but worry about objective data rather than positive individual results. The subject's safety is a priority, but the mission is evaluating the efficacy of medicines and reporting the results precisely. The participant's role is to report the positive and negative effects of the study drug and to share these results.

Clinical trial advertising is complex. Buying advertisements to recruit subjects seems easy, but it is expensive and sometimes wasteful. The message must get to the target group and clearly describes qualifications for taking part in the study. The first step is to pinpoint the media best able to relay the message. The next step is to figure out what group of possible subjects the media are likely to reach. Then deduce what would motivate them to come to the site. Finally, estimate what the media needed to reach that audience is going to cost. Broadcast media, newspapers, neighborhood bulletins, social networking sites, and Internet advertising are the leading choices to consider.

As time goes on, tactics for reaching likely participants will become increasingly refined. Digital medical records may play a leading role. For now, the most difficult problem in health information management is connecting patients to their scattered records. For various reasons, providers doggedly protect their patients' health information. HIPPA makes records even more difficult to get. When health delivery records are fragmented, data from past events may be impossible to get. To make matters worse, insurance may pay patients' claims only if the doctor makes a certain diagnosis or stresses particular key symptoms over others. This practice muddles the use of medical records for confirmation of diagnosis for clinical trials. Finally, medical systems do not talk to one another or even hold similar patient data. New digital records vow to promote cross talk, enabling them to work together. These efforts transform collection, indexing, and distribution of records. Once records precisely link to one another, an accurate picture of a patient's medical history will be available. How clinical trials in the future might use digital records remains unknown; but the database will grow and provide new openings for identifying subjects.

Consent

FDA requires ethics boards to make sure that advertising is accurate. The consent discussion starts before the first contact. Advertising for subjects is the beginning of consent and subject selection. Advertisements should be easy to compare with the approved consent document. Rules that apply when getting a formal consent apply to recruitment. Subjects must fully grasp the effects of taking part, which embraces the benefits, risks, the intent of the study, and the research design. The consent form usually spells this out in a list of choices that includes other treatments and the choice of starting medication immediately. The staff need to discuss all available forms of medical care with the subject. They need to outline the study requirements. For proper recruitment, staff must be certain that subjects are aware of risks and benefits. The study assigns some subjects to take an inert substance and others to active drug. Both researchers and subjects are blind to which participants are taking active drug. Subjects should know that they might get worse if the study asks them to suspend existing treatments that may be working. If a current therapy works, sites must tell subjects about harm that could come from delaying treatment. Subjects must have a chance to respond and ask questions. A simple fact sheet and a pre-consent quiz are helpful. A thorough review is essential, even if some people decide to decline the offer to take part. An unintended benefit is the review helps exclude people who are unlikely to finish the study. At the end, the participant and the researcher sign the consent form. A valid consent must be voluntary, needing the person to understand the risks and benefits as well as the time and effort involved (Carpenter *et al.*, 2003; Michels, 1999).

One of the investigator's chief duties is to make sure subjects give valid consent. People with mental disorders may not recognize what it means to join a study because they have poor emotional control or serious cognitive problems. Consent is continuing and the site assesses the participant's feelings during the whole trial. The team must regularly gauge the subjects' wish to continue. Staff should be sure that subjects know what the study needs to learn. The subject has a critical role in judging the medication and staff ought to reinforce that role constantly.

Project marketing tool kit

Sample project review card

Illness: one line description of the illness

Age:

Birth control status:

Time requirements:

Special considerations:

Sample project review card
Prior participation exclusion:
Acuity:
Medications disallowed:
Concurrent illnesses disallowed:
Caregiver involvement:
Environmental needs:
Substance use exclusions:
Reimbursement if any:

The benefits and obstacles must deliver a compact message. The message must always include a mention that taking part may lead to improved treatment for other people who also have the participant's illness.

Primary marketing tasks

Community outreach
1. Identify key stakeholders and gatekeepers
2. Understand the needs of the stakeholders
3. Develop the message
4. Deliver the message
5. Track performance
Print media
1. Obtain or develop the advertisement
2. Ensure IRB approval
3. Develop a cost-effective delivery strategy
Airwaves
1. Develop or obtain the advertisements
2. Get approvals
3. Determine appropriate media runs based on past performance (detail is important)
4. Track performance of the advertisement
Internet
1. Develop web landing page
2. Research web optimization
3. Track results

Community outreach

Social media campaign

1. Facebook

2. Twitter

3. YouTube

Public relations

1. Press release, public radio, local TV news

Direct mail

1. Get local pharmacies to mail flier

2. Professional associations mail to physicians and other professionals

Email

1. Previous participant newsletter

2. Lists from various organizations

3. Professional email marketers

Training

Indication training for site staff

- PI direct lectures
- Assigned reading material
- Multimedia presentations
- Tests of knowledge

Protocol training for site staff

- Constant review and rehearsal

Marketing training

- Telephone script written by coordinator
- Telephone script approved by IRB
- Telephone script delivered in rehearsal
- Telephone script delivered with supervision to caller
- Telephone script quality assurance

References

(1999). A word from clinical trials volunteers. *Center Watch*, 6.

Adams, C. P. and Brantner, V. V. (2006). Estimating the cost of new drug development: is it really 802 million dollars? *Health Aff (Millwood)*, 25 (2), 420–8.

Armstrong, D. (2008). Doctor didn't disclose Glaxo payments, senator says. *Wall Street Journal*. New York, Dow Jones: A12.

Bain, L. J. (2005). Crossroads in clinical trials. *NeuroRx*, 2 (3), 525–8.

Bentley, J. P. and Thacker, P. G. (2004). The influence of risk and monetary payment on the research participation decision making process. *J Med Ethics*, 30 (3), 293–8.

Bodenheimer, T. (2000). Uneasy alliance — clinical investigators and the pharmaceutical industry. *New Engl J Med*, 342 (20), 1539–44.

Carpenter, W. T., Jr., Appelbaum, P. S., *et al.* (2003). The Declaration of Helsinki and clinical trials: a focus on placebo-controlled trials in schizophrenia. *Am J Psychiat*, 160 (2), 356–62.

DeAngelis, C. D. and Fontanarosa, P. B. (2008). Impugning the integrity of medical science. *J Am Med Assoc*, 299 (15), 1833–5.

Dorsey, E. R., Vitticore, P., *et al.* (2006). Financial anatomy of neuroscience research. *Ann Neurol*, 60 (6), 652–9.

Fava, M., Evins, A. E., *et al.* (2003). The problem of the placebo response in clinical trials for psychiatric disorders: culprits, possible remedies, and a novel study design approach. *Psychother Psychosom*, 72 (3), 115–27.

Getz, K. A., Wenger, J., *et al.* (2008). Assessing the impact of protocol design changes on clinical trial performance. *Am J Ther*, 15 (5), 450–7.

Kaiser, J. (2010). Health bill backs evidence-based medicine, new drug studies. *Science*, 327 (5973), 1562.

Kemp, A. S., Schooler, N. R., *et al.* (2010). What is causing the reduced drug-placebo difference in recent schizophrenia clinical trials and what can be done about it? *Schizophrenia Bull*, 36 (3), 504–9.

Lewis, S. W., Davies, L., *et al.* (2006). Randomised controlled trials of conventional antipsychotic versus new atypical drugs, and new atypical drugs versus clozapine, in people with schizophrenia responding poorly to, or intolerant of, current drug treatment. *Health Technol Assess*, 10 (17), iii–iv, ix–xi, 1–165.

Lexchin, J. (2011). Those who have the gold make the evidence: how the pharmaceutical industry biases the outcomes of clinical trials of medications. *Sci Eng Ethics*, 1–15.

Michels, R. (1999). Are research ethics bad for our mental health? *New Engl J Med*, 340 (18), 1427–30.

Moses, H., Dorsey, III, E. R., *et al.* (2005). Financial anatomy of biomedical research. *J Am Med Assoc*, 294 (11), 1333–42.

Permuth-Wey, J. and Borenstein, A. R. (2009). Financial remuneration for clinical and behavioral research participation: ethical and practical considerations. *Ann Epidemiol*, 19 (4), 280–5.

Sismondo, S. (2008). Pharmaceutical company funding and its consequences: a qualitative systematic review. *Contemporary Clin Trials*, 29 (2), 109–13.

Stiglitz, J. E. and Jayadev, A. (2010). Medicine for tomorrow: some alternative proposals to promote socially beneficial research and development in pharmaceuticals. *J Generic Med*, 7 (3), 217–26.

Targum, S. D. (2006). Evaluating rater competency for CNS clinical trials. *J Clin Psychopharmacol*, 26 (3), 308–10.

Medical writing for CNS indications

Ginette Nachman

Medical writers play an important role in many phases of the clinical drug development process, from initial protocol development to final reporting of clinical trial data. The task of the medical writer is to prepare documents that are unbiased, scientifically and medically accurate, and clearly written. Medical writers often work closely with other project team members, such as medical officers, project managers, regulatory experts, statisticians, and quality control reviewers in document preparation. Because documents have a focus on clinical data presentation and interpretation, medical writers have backgrounds that include training in the biological sciences. Medical writers are individuals who are detail-oriented yet able to step back and see the big picture that emerges from the data and its impact on patient care.

Examples of documents that medical writers prepare include:

- Protocol Outlines, Protocols, and Protocol Amendments
- Investigator Brochures
- Investigational New Drug (IND) Submissions
- Clinical Study Reports (CSRs)
- Abbreviated CSRs
- Patient Narratives for CSRs
- Clinical Trial Registry Reports
- Annual Safety Reports
- Common Technical Document (CTD) Modules
- Briefing Documents
- Manuscripts for publication in professional journals

Most of these documents are prepared for submission to regulatory agencies and must conform to industry standards such as those set by the International Council on Harmonisation (ICH, established in 1990, reflecting input from Europe, Japan, and the United States [US]), or specific regulatory agencies such as the US Food and Drug Administration (FDA) (including applicable guidelines specified in the US Code of Federal Regulations) and the European Medicines Evaluation Agency (EMEA). For example, CSRs are currently expected to conform to ICH E3 guidelines (ICH E3, 1996), which include an outline of sections and topics to be addressed for full CSRs (Table 1). Full CSRs can be quite large (100 to 250 pages in the body of the report and appendices of many thousands of pages). Adherence to standardized approaches ensures that important aspects of inclusion/exclusion criteria, clinical trial design, statistical methodology, and efficacy and safety data are reported uniformly across trials.

Essential CNS Drug Development, ed. A. Kalali, Sheldon Preskorn, J. Kwentus, and Stephen M. Stahl. Published by Cambridge University Press. © Cambridge University Press 2012.

Table 1. ICH E3 Outline for Clinical Study Reports (1996)

1 TITLE PAGE

2 SYNOPSIS

3 TABLE OF CONTENTS

4 LIST OF ABBREVIATIONS AND DEFINITIONS OF TERMS

5 ETHICS

5.1 Independent Ethics Committee (IEC) or Institutional Review Board (IRB)

5.2 Ethical Conduct of the Study

5.3 Patient Information and Consent

6 INVESTIGATORS AND STUDY ADMINISTRATIVE STRUCTURE

7 INTRODUCTION

8 STUDY OBJECTIVES

9 INVESTIGATIONAL PLAN

9.1 Overall Study Design and Plan: Description

9.2 Discussion of Study Design, Including the Choice of Control Groups

9.3 Selection of Study Population

9.3.1 Inclusion Criteria

9.3.2 Exclusion Criteria

9.3.3 Removal of Patients from Therapy or Assessment

9.4 Treatments

9.4.1 Treatments Administered

9.4.2 Identity of Investigational Product(s)

9.4.3 Method of Assigning Patients to Treatment Groups

9.4.4 Selection of Doses in the Study

9.4.5 Selection and Timing of Dose for Each Patient

9.4.6 Blinding

9.4.7 Prior and Concomitant Therapy

9.4.8 Treatment Compliance

9.5 Efficacy and Safety Variables

9.5.1 Efficacy and Safety Measurements Assessed and Flow Chart

9.5.2 Appropriateness of Measurements

9.5.3 Primary Efficacy Variable(s)

9.5.4 Drug Concentration Measurements

9.6 Data Quality Assurance

Table 1. (*cont.*)

9.7 Statistical Methods Planned in the Protocol and Determination of Sample Size

9.7.1 Statistical and Analytical Plans

9.7.2 Determination of Sample Size

9.8 Changes in the Conduct of the Study or Planned Analyses

10 STUDY PATIENTS

10.1 Disposition of Patients

10.2 Protocol Deviations

11 EFFICACY EVALUATION

11.1 Data Sets Analyzed

11.2 Demographic and Other Baseline Characteristics

11.3 Measurements of Treatment Compliance

11.4 Efficacy Results and Tabulations of Individual Patient Data

11.4.1 Analysis of Efficacy

11.4.2 Statistical/Analytical Issues

11.4.2.1 Adjustments for Covariates

11.4.2.2 Handling of Dropouts or Missing Data

11.4.2.3 Interim Analyses and Data Monitoring

11.4.2.4 Multicenter Studies

11.4.2.5 Multiple Comparisons/Multiplicity

11.4.2.6 Use of an "Efficacy Subset" of Patients

11.4.2.7 Active-Control Studies Intended to Show Equivalence

11.4.2.8 Examination of Subgroups

11.4.3 Tabulation of Individual Response Data

11.4.4 Drug Dose, Drug Concentration, and Relationships to Response

11.4.5 Drug-Drug and Drug-Disease Interactions

11.4.6 By-Patient Displays

11.4.7 Efficacy Conclusions

12 SAFETY EVALUATION

12.1 Extent of Exposure

12.2 Adverse Events

12.2.1 Brief Summary of Adverse Events

12.2.2 Display of Adverse Events

12.2.3 Analysis of Adverse Events

12.2.4 Listing of Adverse Events by Patient

Table 1. (cont.)

12.3 Deaths, Other Serious Adverse Events, and Other Significant Adverse Events

12.3.1 Listing of Deaths, Other Serious Adverse Events, and Other Significant Adverse Events

12.3.1.1 Deaths

12.3.1.2 Other Serious Adverse Events

12.3.1.3 Other Significant Adverse Events

12.3.2 Narratives of Deaths, Other Serious Adverse Events, and Certain Other Significant Adverse Events

12.3.3 Analysis and Discussion of Deaths, Other Serious Adverse Events, and Other Significant Adverse Events

12.4 Clinical Laboratory Evaluation

12.4.1 Listing of Individual Laboratory Measurements by Patient and Each Abnormal Laboratory Value

12.4.2 Evaluation of Each Laboratory Parameter

12.4.2.1 Laboratory Values Over Time

12.4.2.2 Individual Patient Changes

12.4.2.3 Individual Clinically Significant Abnormalities

12.5 Vital Signs, Physical Findings, and Other Observations Related to Safety

12.6 Safety Conclusions

13 DISCUSSION AND OVERALL CONCLUSIONS

14 TABLES, FIGURES, AND GRAPHS REFERRED TO BUT NOT INCLUDED IN THE TEXT

14.1 Demographic Data Summary Figures and Tables

14.2 Efficacy Data Summary Figures and Tables

14.3 Safety Data Summary Figures and Tables

14.3.1 Displays of Adverse Events

14.3.2 Listings of Deaths, Other Serious and Significant Adverse Events

14.3.3 Narratives of Deaths, Other Serious and Certain Other Significant Adverse Events

14.3.4 Abnormal Laboratory Value Listing (each patient)

15 REFERENCE LIST

16 APPENDICES

16.1 Study Information

16.1.1 Protocol and Protocol Amendments

16.1.2 Sample case report form

16.1.3 List of IECs or IRBs and representative written information for patient and sample consent forms

16.1.4 List and description of investigators and other important participants in the study, including brief (one page) CVs or equivalent summaries

16.1.5 Signatures of principal or coordinating investigator(s) or sponsor's responsible medical officer, depending on the regulatory authority's requirement

Table 1. (cont.)

16.1.6 Listing of patients receiving test drug(s)/investigational product(s) from specific batches, where more than one batch was used

16.1.7 Randomization scheme and codes (patient identification and treatment assigned)

16.1.8 Audit certificates (if available)

16.1.9 Documentation of statistical methods

16.1.10 Documentation of inter-laboratory standardization methods and quality assurance procedures if used

16.1.11 Publications based on the study

16.1.12 Important publications referenced in the report

16.2 Patient Data Listings

16.2.1 Discontinued patients

16.2.2 Protocol deviations

16.2.3 Patients excluded from the efficacy analysis

16.2.4 Demographic data

16.2.5 Compliance and/or drug concentration data (if available)

16.2.6 Individual efficacy response data

16.2.7 Adverse event listings (each patient)

16.2.8 Listing of individual laboratory measurements by patient, when required by regulatory authorities

16.3 Case Report Forms (CRFs)

16.3.1 CRFs for deaths, other serious adverse events, and withdrawals for adverse events

16.3.2 Other CRFs submitted

16.4 Individual Patient Data Listings

Along with this general approach, medical writing in the area of CNS drug development is associated with some unique issues. This includes familiarity with the measures typically employed in CNS studies including interpretation of the results, as well as specific safety issues to consider when evaluating data.

Measures employed in CNS studies

Measures employed in CNS studies include diagnostic, efficacy, quality of life (QoL), and safety measures. A brief overview of some commonly employed measures is provided below. For additional information on these and other measures the reader is referred to the references provided at the end of this chapter, including some excellent reviews (Guy, 1976; Sajatovic and Ramirez, 2001; AstraZeneca website).

Diagnostic measures

The gold standard for CNS diagnosis is currently the *Diagnostic and Statistical Manual of Mental Disorders, 4th edition – Text Revision* (DSM-IV TR™) (American Psychiatric

Association, 2000). Version V of this manual is being prepared, with a projected release date of May 2013 (American Psychiatric Association website: www.psych.org/MainMenu/Research/DSMIV/DSMV.aspx).

Other diagnostic measures include structured interviews such as the Structured Clinical Interview for Axis I DSM-IV Disorders (SCID) (First *et al.*, 1995), and the Mini-International Neuropsychiatric Interview (MINI) (Sheehan *et al.*, 1998). In addition, diagnostic measures have been developed that are related to specific indications, such as the Bipolarity Index (BPI, to diagnose bipolar disorder) (Sachs, 2004), the Kiddie-Sads-Present and Lifetime (KSADS-PL, to diagnose Attention-Deficit/Hyperactivity Disorder [ADHD]) (Kaufman *et al.*, 2000), and the CAGE Questionnaire (to diagnose alcohol abuse) (Ewing, 1984).

Efficacy, quality of life, and safety measures

A listing of some representative efficacy measures specific to particular CNS indications is presented in Table 2. A listing of representative QoL and safety measures is presented in Table 3.

Efficacy considerations

The analysis and presentation of efficacy findings is driven by a study's statistical analysis plan, which is prepared by the project statistician(s) with input from the project team prior to locking the clinical database. Typically, findings related to the investigational drug will be compared to those of placebo or a drug already marketed for the indication being studied.

There has been growing attention to the increasing placebo effects noted with some CNS drugs, particularly with regard to antidepressant medications (Walsh *et al.*, 2002). Since the gold standard for determining efficacy is to demonstrate significantly greater improvement over placebo treatment, this is becoming increasingly problematic. Placebo effects have not routinely been a focus for data interpretation, other than as a comparator for active treatment. However, examination of the magnitude of placebo effects may become an additional area to consider when reporting findings.

Safety considerations

Analysis of safety data typically includes attention to:

- adverse events that occur after a subject receives his/her first dose of investigational study medication ("treatment-emergent adverse events" [TEAEs], especially serious TEAEs and TEAEs leading to discontinuation from a study)
- analysis of laboratory findings (especially the incidence of markedly abnormal laboratory values, values that shift from normal at baseline to high or low during the study, or values associated with TEAEs) including attention to findings reflecting liver (alanine transaminase, aspartate transaminase, γ-glutamyl transpeptidase, total bilirubin, direct bilirubin, and alkaline phosphatase) or renal (blood urea nitrogen, creatinine) function
- vital signs data (blood pressure, heart rate, temperature)
- electrocardiogram (ECG) data, and
- physical examination findings.

Table 2. Representative efficacy measures used in CNS studies

Schizophrenia and psychotic disorders

Positive and Negative Syndrome Scale (PANSS) (Kay *et al.*, 1987; Kay *et al.*, 1988)

PANSS subscale scores (Positive Symptom score, Negative Symptom score, General Psychopathology score, Marder Factor scores)

Brief Psychiatric Rating Scale (BPRS) (Overall and Gorham, 1962, 1988)

Bipolar disorder*

Young Mania Rating Scale (YMRS) (Young *et al.*, 1978)

Depression

Hamilton Psychiatric Rating Scale for Depression (HAM-D)** (Hamilton, 1960)

Inventory of Depressive Symptomatology – self report (IDS-SR) (Rush *et al.*, 1986; Rush *et al.*, 1996)

Montgomery-Asberg Depression Rating Scale (MADRS) (Montgomery and Asberg, 1979)

Quick Inventory of Depressive Symptomatology – Self Report (QIDS-SR$_{16}$) (Rush *et al.*, 2003)

Anxiety disorders

Hamilton Rating Scale for Anxiety (HAM-A) (Hamilton, 1959)

Liebowitz Social Anxiety Scale (LSAS) (Liebowitz, 1987)

Obsessive compulsive disorder

Yale-Brown Obsessive Compulsive Scale (YBOCS) (Goodman *et al.*, 1989a,b)

Attention deficit hyperactivity disorder

ADHD-Rating Scale-IV (DuPaul *et al.*, 1998)

Conners' Parent Rating Scale – Revised Short Form (CPRS-R:S) (Conners, 1997; Conners *et al.*, 1998a)

Conners' Teacher Rating Scale – Revised Short Version (CTRS-R) (Conners, 1997; Conners *et al.*, 1998b)

Multiple indications

Clinical Global Impression of Severity (CGI-S) (Guy, 1976)

Clinical Global Impression of Improvement (CGI-I) (Guy, 1976)

Sheehan Disability Scale (SDS) (Sheehan, 1983; Sheehan *et al.*, 1996)

Arizona Sexual Experiences Scale (ASEX) (McGahuey *et al.*, 2000)

Changes in Sexual Functioning Questionnaire (CSFQ) (Clayton *et al.*, 1997)

Columbia Suicide Severity Rating Scale (CSSRS) (Posner *et al.*, 2007)

InterSept Scale for Suicidality (ISST) (Lindenmayer *et al.*, 2003) (for Schizophrenia and Schizoaffective Disorders)

* See depression measures as well.
** 21 item and 17 item versions.

Table 3. Representative quality of life and safety measures used in CNS studies

Quality of life measures

Quality of Life Scale (QLS) (for schizophrenia) (Heinrichs et al., 1984)

Quality of Life Enjoyment and Satisfaction Scale (Q-LES-Q) (Endicott et al., 1993)

Quality of Life Enjoyment and Satisfaction Scale – Short Form (Q-LES-Q-SF) (Schechter et al., 2007)

Personal Evaluations of Transitions and Treatments (PETiT) (Voruganti and Awad, 2002)

Safety measures*

Abnormal Involuntary Movement Scale (AIMS) (see Guy, 1976)

Barnes Akathisia Scale (BAS, BARS) (Barnes, 1989)

Extrapyramidal Symptom Rating Scale (ESRS) (Chouinard et al., 1980)

Simpson Angus Scale (SAS, SARS) (Simpson and Angus, 1970)

Udvalg for Kliniske Undersogelser (UKU) Side Effect Rating Scale (Lingjaerde et al., 1987)

*The most common safety measures used to assess potential side effects of CNS medication are those employed in studies of antipsychotic medication assessing for movement disorder side effects. In addition, measures used to assess suicidality (Table 2) may be reported as safety measures.

Any safety concerns that are noted in pre-clinical or prior clinical studies using the investigational product may also be targeted for specific review. In addition, there are a number of safety issues that are typical to studies involving CNS drugs.

Adverse events of interest in CNS studies generally include TEAEs related to the indication studied (increased anxiety, depression, psychosis, etc.), as well as TEAEs of suicidal/homicidal ideation or attempt. Adverse events related to effects on weight are also often of interest. Weight gain, in particular, has been identified as a factor contributing to poor compliance in patients receiving antipsychotic medication (Tschoner et al., 2007; Weiden et al., 2004) and increased risk for metabolic syndrome. Safety considerations relevant to particular CNS indications are detailed below.

Antipsychotic medications

Antipsychotic medications have been associated with a number of side effects including lethargy, somnolence, dizziness, orthostatic hypotension, extrapyramidal side effects (EPS) (akathisia, dystonia, tremors, parkinsonism), tardive dyskinesia, neuroleptic malignant syndrome, hyperprolactinemia, sexual difficulties, and QT interval prolongation. There has been growing recognition that while newer atypical antipsychotic medications are generally associated with fewer EPS compared with older medications, they are often (to varying degrees depending on the particular medication) associated with more weight gain and metabolic side effects such as diabetes, increases in blood glucose levels, and dyslipidemias (Tschoner et al., 2007, 2009). These latter side effects are associated with a cluster of potential risk factors for cardiovascular disease termed "metabolic syndrome" (McEvoy et al., 2005; Monteleone et al., 2009; Straker et al., 2005). Evaluation of the safety profile of investigational antipsychotic medication typically includes attention to these potential side effects, both to rule out safety issues and to establish possible advantages in the marketplace. We will briefly consider some of these issues and parameters that are typically reviewed during analysis of data.

Metabolic syndrome. Although there has been some variation in the criteria used to define metabolic syndrome, with different definitions proposed, for example, by the National Cholesterol Education Program Adult Treatment Panel (NCEP-ATP) III, the World Health Organization (WHO), and the International Diabetes Federation (IDF), common criteria include "(abdominal) obesity (waist circumference), insulin resistance, dyslipidemia, and hypertension" (Cornier *et al.*, 2008). Given the increasing attention to these metabolic side effects, some studies of antipsychotic medication include an assessment of metabolic syndrome impact using pre-defined criteria. In addition, TEAEs related to increases or decreases in glucose (including new-onset or worsening diabetes), blood pressure, and body weight are reviewed. Laboratory assessment typically includes attention to increases or decreases in glucose, insulin (if assessed), as well as lipid parameters such as low density lipoprotein (LDL), HDL, and triglycerides (with special attention given to shifts to high in LDL or triglycerides, and to some extent, shifts to low in HDL).

Extrapyramidal symptoms. Treatment-emergent adverse events of EPS are always of interest in studies of antipsychotic medication. In addition to evaluating the incidence of tardive dyskinesia, tremor, akathisia, dystonia, and parkinsonism, medical writers may also assess relative usage of concomitant medications such as benztropine, biperiden, diphenhydramine, and trihexyphenidyl, used to treat these events. Measures such as the SAS, BAS, and AIMS (Table 3) are also commonly employed in the assessment of EPS side effects.

Neuroleptic malignant syndrome. Neuroleptic malignant syndrome (NMS) is a rare but potentially life-threatening disorder associated with the use of antipsychotic medications. First noted with older typical antipsychotic medications (Delay *et al.*, 1960), it has also been observed with newer atypical medications (Trollor *et al.*, 2009). The disorder is characterized by "fever, severe muscle rigidity, autonomic, and mental status changes" (Strawn *et al.*, 2007). Elevated serum creatine kinase and other abnormalities including "impaired liver function tests, leucocytosis, electrolyte disturbance, renal impairment, altered coagulation studies, and ECG abnormalities" (Trollor *et al.*, 2009) have also been associated with the condition. Given their potential severity, TEAEs of NMS are always of interest in studies of antipsychotic medication.

Hyperprolactinemia. Hyperprolactinemia has been associated with older antipsychotic medications as well as some newer atypical medications. While often not associated with obvious adverse effects, potential health consequences can include amenorrhea or menstrual irregularities, galactorrhea, gynecomastia, and sexual dysfunctions such as loss of libido or fertility, orgasmic dysfunction, prolonged erection, or priapism (Monteleone *et al.*, 2009). Other potential long-term problems may include osteoporosis, increased risk of breast or endometrial cancer, and insulin resistance, although more research is needed in these areas (Monteleone *et al.*, 2009). The incidence of TEAEs related to these issues (particularly short-term effects), in subjects known to have hyperprolactinemia, is often of interest in studies of antipsychotic medication.

QT prolongation. The QT interval on an ECG represents the interval between onset of the QRS complex and completion of the T wave, and largely reflects ventricular repolarization (Vieweg *et al.*, 2009). Because the QT interval varies inversely with heart rate, it is typically corrected using either the Bazett (QTcB) or Fridericia (QTcF) correction.

Prolongation of the QT interval has been associated with a dangerous arrhythmia known as polymorphic ventricular tachycardia (and its subtype, torsade de pointes). Polymorphic ventricular tachycardia can lead to sudden cardiac death, and has been associated with some antipsychotic and antidepressant medications. Given the association of QT prolongation with some CNS medications, assessment of QT prolongation is included in clinical trials of CNS medications. Study-specific assessment of QT prolongation may vary somewhat, but a typical definition is: QTcB $\geq$450 ms (men) and QTcB $\geq$470 ms (women) (Goldenberg et al., 2006). Along with attention to possible QT prolongation, medical writers attend to the incidence of abnormal arrhythmias and other reported clinically significant ECG abnormalities as well as related TEAEs/serious TEAEs.

Antidepressant medications

Along with issues related to sedation, possible QT prolongation, and weight changes (loss or gain depending on medication), a negative impact on sexual functioning has been associated with several antidepressant medications and has received increasing attention in the literature. Depression itself is associated with an increased incidence of sexual dysfunction which can be further exacerbated by antidepressant medications. Although differences exist depending on particular medications, many antidepressant medications have been associated with reduced sexual desire, arousal difficulties including erectile dysfunction, and orgasmic dysfunction including problems with ejaculation. These sexual side effects in turn can increase feelings of depression. Sexual adverse effects have been recognized as a major source of medication non-compliance and treatment discontinuation in patients receiving antidepressant medication (Kennedy and Rizvi, 2009; Schweitzer et al., 2009). Attention to TEAEs related to sexual difficulties is therefore an important consideration when evaluating data related to antidepressant medication. In addition, it should be noted that some antidepressant medications such as selective serotonin reuptake inhibitors (known to be associated with sexual dysfunction; Corona et al., 2009) are also prescribed for other psychiatric conditions including anxiety disorders (Schweitzer et al., 2009).

Finally, it has been recognized that some individuals who initially demonstrate a good response to a particular antidepressant treatment may stop responding to that treatment over time (Leib and Balter, 1984). This effect, termed "antidepressant tachyphylaxis", is also important to consider when reporting long-term studies of antidepressant medication.

Current trends in medical writing for CNS indications

In recent years, medical writing has been influenced by two major related trends: a trend towards increased standardization and a trend towards increased efficiency in the production of documents. Increased standardization is reflected in the recent change to the common technical document (CTD) format for new drug submissions, and adherence to ICH E3 guidelines for CSRs. Increased efficiency is reflected in the change from paper to electronic submission of regulatory documents. A major advantage of electronic submissions is the inclusion of electronic hyperlinks that can facilitate review by linking text to supporting documentation. Given increasing pressure to shorten deliverable timelines, and the ease of accessing relevant data through such hyperlinks, it is possible that regulatory documents of the future will move to briefer summary formats with less reliance on in-text tabular summaries of data.

References

American Psychiatric Association. (2000). *Diagnostic and Statistical Manual of Mental Disorders, 4th edition, Text Revision.* Washington DC, APA.

American Psychiatric Association website: http://www.psych.org/MainMenu/Research/DSMIV/DSMV.aspx (Accessed 03 January 2010).

AstraZeneca website (www.seroquel.info/assessment-tools/).

Barnes, T. R. (1989). A rating scale for drug-induced akathisia. *Brit J Pharmacol*, 154, 672–6.

Chouinard, G., Ross-Chouinard, A., Annable, L., *et al.* (1980). Extrapyramidal Symptom Rating Scale. *Can J Neurol Sci*, 7, 233.

Clayton, A. H., McGarvey, E. L., and Clavet, G. J. (1997). The Changes in Sexual Functioning Questionnaire (CSFQ): development, reliability, and validity. *Psychopharmacol Bull*, 33 (4), 731–45.

Conners, C. K. (1997). *Manual for the Conners' Rating Scales – Revised.* North Tonawanda, NY: Multi-Health Systems.

Conners, C. K., Sitarenios, G., Parker, J. D., *et al.* (1998a). The revised Conners' Parent Rating Scale (CPRS-R): factor structure, reliability and criterion validity. *J Abnorm Child Psych*, 26 (4), 257–68.

Conners, C. K., Sitarenios, G., Parker, J. D., *et al.* (1998b). Revision and restandardization of the Conners Teacher Rating Scale (CTRS-R): factor structure, reliability, and criterion validity. *J Abnorm Child Psych*, 26 (4), 279–91.

Cornier, M.-A., Dabelea, D., Hernandez, T. L., *et al.* (2008). The metabolic syndrome. *Endocr Rev*, 29 (7), 777–822.

Corona, G., Ricca, V., Bandini, E., *et al.* (2009). Selective serotonin reuptake inhibitor-induced sexual dysfunction. *J Sex Med*, 6, 1259–69.

Delay, J., Pichot, P., Lemperiere, T., *et al.* (1960). A non-phenothiazine and non-reserpine major neuroleptic, haloperidol, in the treatment of psychoses. *Ann Med Psychol (Paris)*, 118 (1), 145–52.

DuPaul, G. J., Power, T. J., Anastopoulos, A. D., *et al.* (1998). *ADHD Rating Scale-IV: Checklists, normals, and clinical interpretation.* New York: Guilford Press.

Endicott, J., Nee, J., Harrison, W., and Blumenthal, R. (1993). Quality of Life Enjoyment and Satisfaction Questionnaire: a new measure. *Psychopharmacol Bull*, 29, 321–6.

Ewing, J. A. (1984). Detecting alcoholism: the CAGE Questionnaire. *J Am Med Assoc*, 252 (14), 1905–7.

First, M. B., Spitzer, R. L., Gibbon, M., *et al.* (1995). *Structured Clinical Interview for DSM-IV Axis I Disorders.* New York, NY: State Psychiatric Institute, Biometrics Research.

Goldenberg, I., Moss, A. J., and Zareba, W. (2006). QT interval: how to measure it and what is "normal". *J Cardiovasc Electrophysiol*, 17, 333–6.

Goodman, W. K., Price, L. H., Rasmussen, S. A., *et al.* (1989a). The Yale-Brown Obsessive Compulsive Scale I: development, use, and reliability. *Arch Gen Psychiat*, 46 (11), 1006–11.

Goodman, W. K., Price, L. H., Rasmussen, S. A., *et al.* (1989b). The Yale-Brown Obsessive Compulsive Scale II: validity. *Arch Gen Psychiat*, 46 (11), 1012–16.

Guy, W. (1976). *ECDEU Assessment Manual for Psychopharmacology, Revised 1976.* Rockville (MD): (NIMH) National Institute of Mental Health, Psychopharmacology Research Branch.

Hamilton, M. (1959). The assessment of anxiety states by rating. *Br J Med Psychol*, 32, 50–5.

Hamilton, M. (1960). A rating scale for depression. *J Neurol Neurosurg Psy*, 23, 56–62.

Heinrichs, D. W., Hanlon, T. E., and Carpenter, W. T. (1984). Quality of Life scale: an instrument for rating the schizophrenic deficit scale. *Schizophrenia Bull*, 10, 388–98.

ICH E3 Guideline for Industry: Structure and Content of Clinical Study Reports, July 1996.

Kaufman, J., Birmaher, B., Brent, D. A., *et al.* (2000). K-SADS-PL. *J Am Acad Child Adolesc Psychiatr*, 39 (1), 49–58.

Kay, S. R., Fiszbein, A., and Opler, L. A. (1987). The Positive and Negative Syndrome Scale (PANSS) for schizophrenia. *Schizophrenia Bull*, 13, 261–76.

Kay, S. R., Opler, L. A., and Lindenmayer, J. P. (1988). Reliability and validity of the Positive and Negative Syndrome Scale for schizophrenics. *Psychiat Res*, 23, 99–110.

Kennedy, S. H. and Rizvi, S. (2009). Sexual dysfunction, depression, and the impact of antidepressants. *J Clinic Psychopharmacol*, 29 (2), 157–64.

Lieb, J. and Balter, A. (1984). Antidepressant tachyphylaxis. *Med Hypotheses*, 15 (3), 279–91.

Liebowitz, M. R. (1987). Social phobia. *Mod Probl Pharmacopsychiat*, 22, 141–73.

Lindenmayer, J. P., Czobor, P., Alphs, L., *et al.* (2003). The InterSePT scale for suicidal thinking reliability and validity. *Schizophrenia Res*, 63, 161–70.

Lingjaerde, O., Ahlfors, U. G., Bech, P., *et al.* (1987). The UKU Side Effect Rating Scale. A new comprehensive rating scale for psychotropic drugs and a cross-sectional study of side effects in neuroleptic-treated patients. *Acta Psychiatr Scand Suppl*, 334, 1–100.

McEvoy, J., Meyer, J., Goff, D., *et al.* (2005). Prevalence of the metabolic syndrome in patients with schizophrenia: baseline results from the clinical antipsychotic trials of intervention effectiveness (CATIE) schizophrenia trial and comparison with national estimates from NHANES III. *Schizophrenia Res*, 66 (1), 19–32.

McGahuey, C. A., Gelenberg, A. J., Laukes, C. A., *et al.* (2000). The Arizona Sexual Experiences Scale (ASEX): reliability and validity. *J Sex Marital Ther*, 26 (1), 25–40.

Monteleone, P., Martiadis, V., and Maj, M. (2009). Management of schizophrenia with obesity, metabolic, and endocrinological disorders. *Psychiat Clin N Am*, 32 (4), 775–94.

Montgomery, S. A. and Asberg, M. (1979). A new depression scale designed to be sensitive to change. *Brit J Psychiat*, 134, 382–9.

Overall, J. E. and Gorham, D. R. (1962). The Brief Psychiatric Rating Scale. *Psychol Rep*, 10, 799–812.

Overall, J. E. and Gorham, D. R. (1988). The Brief Psychiatric Rating Scale: recent developments in ascertainment and scaling. *Psychopharmacol Bull*, 24, 97–9.

Posner, K., Melvin, G. A., Stanley, B., *et al.* (2007). Factors in the assessment of suicidality in youth. *CNS Spectr*, 12, 156–62.

Rush, A. J., Giles, D. E., Schlesser, M. A., *et al.* (1986). The Inventory of Depressive Symptomatology (IDS): preliminary findings. *Psychiat Res*, 18, 65–87.

Rush, A. J., Gullion, C. M., Basco, M. R., *et al.* (1996). The Inventory of Depressive Symptomatology (IDS): psychometric properties. *Psychol Med*, 26, 477–86.

Rush, A. J., Trivedi, M. H., Ibrahim, H. M., *et al.* (2003). The 16-Item Quick Inventory of Depressive Symptomatology (QIDS), clinician rating (QIDS-C), and self report (QIDS-SR): a psychometric evaluation in patients with chronic major depression. *Biol Psychiat*, 54 (5), 573–83.

Sachs, G. S. (2004). Strategies for improving treatment of bipolar disorder: integration of measurement and management. *Acta Psychiatr Scand Suppl*, 422, 7–17.

Sajatovic, M. and Ramirez, L. F. (2001). *Rating Scales in Mental Health*. Hudson, OH: Lexi-Comp Inc.

Schechter, D., Endicott, J., and Nee, J. (2007). Quality of life of 'normal' controls: association with lifetime history of mental illness. *Psychiat Res*, 152, 45–54.

Schweitzer, I., Maguire, K., and Ng, C. (2009). Sexual side-effects of contemporary antidepressants: review. *Aust NZ J Psychiat*, 43, 795–808.

Sheehan, D. V. (1983). *The Anxiety Disease*. New York: Scribner's.

Sheehan, D. V., Lecrubier, Y., Harnett, Sheehan K., *et al.* (1998). The Mini-International Neuropsychiatric Interview (M.I.N.I.): the development and validation of a structured diagnostic psychiatric interview for DSM-IV and ICD-10. *Journal of Clinical Psychiatry*, 59 (Suppl 20), 22–57.

Sheehan, D. V., Harnett-Sheehan, K., and Raj, B. A. (1996). The measurement of disability. *Int Clin Psychopharmacol*, 11 (suppl 3), 89–95.

Simpson, G. N. and Angus, J. W. S. (1970). A rating scale for extrapyramidal side effects. *Acta Psychiatr Scand Suppl*, 212, 11–19.

Straker, D., Correll, C. U., Kramer-Ginsberg, E., *et al.* (2005). Cost effective screening for the metabolic syndrome in patients treated with second-generation antipsychotic medications. *Am J Psychiat*, 162, 1217–21.

Strawn, J. R., Keck, P. E. Jr, and Caroff, S. N. (2007). Neuroleptic malignant syndrome. *Am J Psychiat*, 164 (6), 870–6.

Trollor, J. N., Chen, X., and Sachdev, P. S. (2009). Neuroleptic malignant syndrome associated with atypical antipsychotic drugs. *CNS Drugs*, 23 (6), 477–92.

Tschoner, A., Engl, J., Laimer, M., *et al.* (2007). Metabolic side effects of antipsychotic medication. *Int J Clin Pract*, 61 (8), 1356–70.

Tschoner, A., Fleischhacker, W. W., and Ebenbichler, C. F. (2009). Experimental antipsychotics and metabolic adverse effects – findings from clinical trials. *Curr Opin Investigational Drugs*, 10 (10), 1041–8.

Vieweg, W. V., Wood, M. A., Fernandez, A., *et al.* (2009). Proarrythmic risk with antipsychotic and antidepressant drugs: implications in the elderly. *Drugs Aging*, 26 (12), 997–1012.

Voruganti, L. N. P. and Awad, A. G. (2002). Personal Evaluation of Transitions in Treatment (PETiT): a scale to measure subjective aspects of antipsychotic drug therapy in schizophrenia. *Schizophrenia Res*, 56, 37–46.

Walsh, B. T., Seidman, S. N., Sysko, R., and Gould, M. (2002). Placebo response in studies of major depression: variable, substantial, and growing. *J Am Med Assoc*, 287 (14), 1840–7.

Weiden, P. J., Mackell, J. A., and McDonnell, D. D. (2004). Obesity as a risk factor for antipsychotic noncompliance. *Schizophrenia Res*, 66, 51–7.

Young, R. C., Biggs, J. T., Siegler, V. E., *et al.* (1978). A rating scale for mania: reliability, validity, and sensitivity. *Brit J Psychiat*, 133, 429–35.

Dissemination of clinical trial information: multiple audiences, multiple formats

Leslie Citrome

Disclosures

No writing assistance was utilized in the production of this chapter. Within the last 12 months Leslie Citrome was a consultant for, has received honoraria from, or has conducted clinical research supported by the following: AstraZeneca Pharmaceuticals, Bristol-Myers Squibb, Eli Lilly and Company, Janssen Pharmaceuticals, Merck, Novartis, Noven Pharmaceuticals, Pfizer Inc, Shire, Sunovion, and Valeant Pharmaceuticals.

Before the research gets done

The dissemination of clinical trial information has become more transparent and now begins with protocol registration in publicly accessible registries. Following the lead of the International Committee of Medical Journal Editors, many medical journals have begun to require registration of clinical trials as a condition for publication for "any research study that prospectively assigns human participants or groups of humans to one or more health-related interventions to evaluate the effects on health outcomes" (ICMJE). The US National Library of Medicine has developed a registry (clinicaltrials.gov) where the general public can access information posted prior to patient enrollment regarding key study elements such as sponsor, purpose, study population, interventions to be tested, study design, and the primary outcome measure(s). Registry entries can also have hypertext links to other resources, and once the study is complete can also contain a summary of results. Greater attention is being paid to the registry entries and the pre-specified primary outcome measures, and whether or not the study reports as published maintain consistency with what had been disclosed (Mathieu *et al.*, 2009).

For novel methodologies it is becoming more common to see the publication of the protocols well before the study has been completed. This includes the Clinical Antipsychotic Trials of Intervention Effectiveness (CATIE) for schizophrenia (Stroup *et al.*, 2003) and a series of studies designed to test the treatment of negative symptoms of schizophrenia with asenapine (Alphs *et al.*, 2007). Of note, it is routine practice for meta-analyses published by the Cochrane Collaboration to be preceded by a published protocol.

Immediately after the preliminary results are available

Press releases, often in conjunction with the announcement that results will be presented at a national or international scientific meeting, are also used to disseminate study outcomes that may have substantial public health importance or are key to the

Essential CNS Drug Development, ed. A. Kalali, Sheldon Preskorn, J. Kwentus, and Stephen M. Stahl. Published by Cambridge University Press. © Cambridge University Press 2012.

development of a new therapeutic agent. Press releases are also intended to inform potential investors who have been closely following the progress of a specific line of investigation.

Dissemination of results to outside researchers first takes place at scientific meetings. Scientific meetings or congresses usually have provisions for posters and/or oral presentations for new research, and some venues have the capacity to include late-breaking developments, with submission deadlines well after the more routine applications. Although handouts at oral presentations are not the norm, poster miniatures are expected by attendees at poster sessions and some organizations make these available on-line to conference attendees. The abstracts themselves are in the conference proceedings books, with some published as supplements to journals and indexed using services such as Elsevier Embase.

Publication

Although publication in a medical journal is thought to be a definitive record of the results, on-line registries for results, either within protocol registries such as clinicaltrials.gov or in separately maintained resources such as www.clinicalstudyresults.org or those maintained by individual firms, such as http://www.bms.com/clinical_trials/results, can disseminate results well in advance of journal publication. This may be an issue with the editorial policies of some journals regarding prior publication, and will need to be discussed in advance of submission with the journal staff if applicable.

Best practices for publication have been debated and published, with the most recent resources being the Good Publication Practice (GPP2) guidelines (Graf *et al.*, 2009), and the Medical Publishing Insights and Practices (MPIP) initiative (Chipperfield *et al.*, 2010; Clark *et al.*, 2010). Table 1 outlines what is described in the MPIP initiative's Authors' Submission Toolkit (Chipperfield *et al.*, 2010). Aside from the CONSORT guidelines (Schulz *et al.*, 2010), others are available that will help standardize the reporting of results and are well summarized by the Enhancing the Quality and Transparency of Health Research (EQUATOR) network's website and additional resources are outlined in Table 2.

Journal selection has become more complex. The internet has become the great equalizer in terms of accessibility of a study report, provided that the report has been published in a journal that is indexed through the National Library of Medicine's PubMed database. Publishing in a journal with a high impact factor will not necessarily guarantee extensive dissemination (Citrome, 2007), but it may influence how readily the paper is picked up by the news aggregators that report on the latest publications (Citrome *et al.*, 2009). Although there are no obstacles in obtaining abstracts, the open-access model of publishing will eliminate any cost barriers that may exist in obtaining the complete report.

After the principal results are published

Once the principal paper has been published, ancillary and post hoc analyses will help place the original results into clinical perspective. Reviews are also a good opportunity to reiterate the main findings of original studies and provide a means to integrate a body of evidence into a meaningful context. Although sponsored supplements have received negative attention in terms of accusations of bias and lack of objectivity, papers in supplements can be quite influential and highly cited (Citrome, 2010a).

Table 1. Authors' Submission Toolkit contents (Chipperfield *et al.*, 2010)

1. Before the study and writing begin

    a. Authorship and contributorship

        i. Stakeholder roles

        ii. Contributions from professional medical writers, agencies, or sponsors

        iii. Corresponding author

        iv. Publication charter

    b. Conflict of interest disclosures

    c. Prior presentation and publication policies

    d. Understanding the publication plan

    e. Other issues prior to beginning a study

        i. Journal instructions and resources

        ii. Appropriate design

        iii. Reporting requirements from regulators

        iv. Guidelines on reporting research

2. Journal selection

    a. Step 1: conduct an internal assessment

        i. Who do I want to reach (target audience)?

        ii. How do I intend to reach the desired audience?

        iii. How will readers access my article?

        iv. What type of journal will best meet my needs?

        v. How soon do I want or need to publish the data?

    b. Step 2: research journal options

    c. Step 3: identify top choices

3. Publishing research findings of "specialized interest"

4. Pre-submission inquiries

    a. Importance of the pre-submission inquiry

    b. Completing a pre-submission inquiry

5. Manuscript preparation

    a. Important considerations

        i. Adherence to journal's instructions

        ii. Grammar, punctuation, language

        iii. Internal consistency

        iv. Transparency

        v. Author approval

Table 1. (cont.)

b. Best practices by manuscript section

    i. Title and abstract

    ii. Acknowledgments

    iii. Introduction

    iv. Methods

    v. Results

    vi. Discussion

    vii. Conclusion

    viii. References

6. Cover letters

a. Purpose

b. Key elements

7. Review, revision, and re-submission

a. Understanding the review process

b. Best practices in revision and re-submission

c. Defining next steps following a rejection

Regulatory documents as a source of information

The product label as approved by regulatory authorities contains information on clinical trial results, and for some studies on newly approved agents the product label may be the only public source of this information. Product labels can be mined for additional information to make indirect comparisons between competing agents (Citrome, 2009; Citrome and Nasrallah, in press). Briefing documents and Drug Approval Packages can also be sources of information about clinical trials. These documents are in the public domain and accessible to researchers (Citrome, 2010b).

Getting the word out: CME and other educational programs

Continuing medical education (CME) is an important component in the dissemination of study results to clinicians in the field. The incorporation of new findings into educational presentations generally occurs when the results have been generally well disseminated amongst other researchers and educators. Overinterpretation of study results can be a cause for concern and at times mistakes are made at this stage because the persons involved in producing the educational materials may not have all the information available regarding protocol design and the actual conduct of the study. The most valued of CME programs are those that are accredited for category I credits (Accreditation Council for Continuing Medical Education), of which a certain number are required annually for the maintenance of hospital privileges and in many cases, state licensure to practice medicine.

Table 2. On-line resources regarding standards and guidance

1. American Medical Writers Association (AMWA). Available at: http://www.amwa.org/

2. ASSERT (A Standard for the Scientific and Ethical Review of Trials) initiative. Available at: http://www.assert-statement.org/

3. Committee on Publication Ethics (COPE). Available at: http://publicationethics.org/

4. CONSORT Statement 2010. Available at: http://www.consort-statement.org/

5. Council of Science Editors. White Paper on Promoting Integrity in Scientific Journal Publications, 2009 Update. Available at: http://www.councilscienceeditors.org/editorial_policies/whitepaper/entire_whitepaper.pdf

6. Directory of Open Access Journals. Available at: http://www.doaj.org/

7. European Medicines Agency (EMA) Good Clinical Practice. Available at: http://www.ema.europa.eu/Inspections/GCPgeneral.html

8. International Society for Medical Publication Professionals. Available at: http://www.ismpp.org/

9. Jacobs A, Wager E. European Medical Writers Association (EMWA) guidelines on the role of medical writers in developing peer-reviewed publications. CMRO 2005; 21(2):317–21. Available at http://www.emwa.org/MembersDocs/GuidelinesCMRO.pdf

10. EQUATOR (Enhancing the Quality and Transparency of Health Research) Network. Available at: http://www.equator-network.org/

11. European Medical Writers Association (EMWA). Available at: http://www.emwa.org/

12. Food and Drug Administration Amendments Act (FDAAA) of 2007. Available at: http://www.fda.gov/RegulatoryInformation/Legislation/FederalFoodDrugandCosmeticActFDCAct/SignificantAmendmentstotheFDCAct/FoodandDrugAdministrationAmendmentsActof2007/default.htm

13. International Committee of Medical Journal Editors (ICMJE). Uniform Requirements for Manuscripts Submitted to Biomedical Journals: Writing and Editing for Biomedical Publications. Available at: http://www.icmje.org/

14. Medical Publishing Insights and Practices initiative. Available at: http://www.mpip-initiative.org/

15. Stroup DF, Berlin JA, Morton SC, *et al*. Meta-analysis of observational studies in epidemiology: a proposal for reporting. Meta-analysis Of Observational Studies in Epidemiology (MOOSE) group. JAMA 2000; 283(15):2008–2012. Available at: http://jama.ama-assn.org/cgi/reprint/283/15/2008

16. PRISMA (Preferred Reporting Items for Systematic Reviews and Meta-Analyses) Statement (previously the QUOROM Statement). Available at: http://www.prisma-statement.org/

17. STARD (Standards for the Reporting of Diagnostic Accuracy Studies) Statement. Available at: http://www.stard-statement.org/

18. STROBE (Strengthening the Reporting of Observational Studies in Epidemiology) Statement. Available at: http://www.strobe-statement.org/

19. World Medical Association (WMA). Declaration of Helsinki – Ethical Principles for Medical Research Involving Human Subjects Declaration of Helsinki (2008). Available at: http://www.wma.net/en/30publications/10policies/b3/index.html

20. World Health Organization (WHO). International Clinical Trials Registry Platform (ICTRP). Available at: http://www.who.int/ictrp/en/

21. World Health Organization (WHO). Regional Publications Eastern Mediterranean Series 30 – A Practical Guide for Health Researchers. Available at: http://whqlibdoc.who.int/emro/2004/9290213639.pdf

Table 3. Effect size measures

Effect size	Value for no difference	Value for largest possible effect (theoretical)	Typical example of a small effect	Typical example of a large effect
Relative measures				
Relative risk	1	∞	2	4
Odds ratio	1	∞	2	4
Hazard ratio	1	∞	2	4
Absolute measures				
Attributable risk	0	100%	<10%	33–50%
Number needed to treat	∞	1	≥10	2–3
Cohen's *d*	0	∞	0.2	0.8
Area under the curve	0.50	1.00	0.56	0.71
Success rate difference	0	1	0.11	0.43

Adapted from Citrome, 2010c.

Promotional programming in the US, as regulated by the Food and Drug Administration Division of Drug Marketing, Advertising, and Communications, can play a limited role in the discussion of clinical trial outcomes. Content regarding the specific intervention in question is restricted to essentially what is contained in the product label and speakers are held to the same requirements as for the content of TV and radio advertisements, and all written or printed prescription drug promotional materials. Different regulations apply to other countries where pharmaceutical companies can directly engage in educational activities that are often indistinguishable from accredited CME programs found in the USA.

Presenting results – a caveat

Although great effort is made to demonstrate statistical superiority of one intervention versus another (including placebo), insufficient attention is paid regarding the clinical relevance or clinical significance of the outcomes. Obtaining a *P*-value of less than 0.05 becomes the goal in order to have a paper to be of interest to journal editors and deemed worthy of publication (Citrome, Call for papers). This can lead readers astray as it ignores the importance of effect size in appraising results. The effect size of a treatment represents how large a clinical response is observed (Citrome, 2008, 2010c; Kraemer and Kupfer, 2006). Table 3 lists commonly used effect size measures. For continuous outcome measures such as point change on a rating scale, the effect size can be standardized so that it is easier to compare treatment effects in a meta-analysis. For categorical outcomes such as whether or not response or remission was achieved, proportions can be directly compared by simple subtraction to calculate the effect size difference. The reciprocal of this difference in proportions is the "number needed to treat" (NNT), a number that is clinically intuitive and helps relate the effect size difference back to the realities of clinical practice. Number needed to harm (NNH) is used to describe an outcome that is undesirable.

Emerging and non-English-speaking markets

Emerging markets hold special challenges for the dissemination of clinical trial results. Although there is greater clinical trial activity in these countries, not all specialties are at the same level of development.

From the point of view of a medical journal located in an emerging market, access to resources may differ, and governmental or professional society sponsorship may be essential for survival, as would indexing in an easily accessible journal article database such as PubMed. Cultural norms may be different from "Western journals"; for example, the role of the Editor-in-Chief may be that of a figurehead with little involvement in the day-to-day operations of the journal.

From the point of view of the clinician practicing in an emerging market, access to the printed literature may be limited, as would be access to new medications, diagnostic tests, or technologically intensive tools. Cultural influences may determine who becomes a physician and when (often earlier in the educational ladder than in the USA), as well as the authority and influence of the academic professor or government official. Acceptance of "Western" medicine is not a given. Access to healthcare may be quite limited for large portions of the population.

Although on-line access to medical information can differ between countries and between practitioners and researchers, the major obstacles to access are probably subscription fees. Here the open-access model will ease dissemination. Translations may be necessary for specific reports for which wide dissemination is desired.

From the point of view of the pharmaceutical company, the demarcation between promotional activities and continuing medical education may be blurred, and difficult to understand for a company accustomed to the regulatory environment extant in the USA.

Summary

The dissemination of clinical research results has gone through several evolutionary steps, almost all of them attributable to the availability of the world-wide web. Registration of protocols prior to enrolling the first patient is now the norm. The rapid dissemination of preliminary results through press releases and oral and poster presentations at national and international congresses is expected for pivotal trials. On-line registries for clinical trial results are now in place, with results disclosed often prior to publication in a medical journal. Medical journals themselves have become simpler to access, and for articles that are published using the open-access model, easily downloadable. The key factor no longer appears to be the Journal Impact Factor, but the journal's membership in an on-line indexing service. Dissemination of clinical trial information doesn't stop with the study report, but continues with secondary publications, reviews, and educational presentations. Best practices include the presentation of information related to clinical relevance, and here effect sizes need to be made explicit, preferably using metrics that clinicians will find intuitive, such as NNT and NNH. Emerging markets hold special challenges related to differences in language, culture, and availability of information and technology.

References

Accreditation Council for Continuing Medical Education. Available at: http://www.accme. org/. Accessed 2 June 2011.

Alphs, L., Panagides, J., and Lancaster, S. (2007). Asenapine in the treatment of negative symptoms of schizophrenia: clinical trial design and rationale. *Psychopharmacol Bull*, 40 (2), 41–53.

Chipperfield, L., Citrome, L., Clark, J., *et al.* (2010). Authors' Submission Toolkit: a practical guide to getting your research published. *Curr Med Res Opin*, 26 (8), 1967–82.

Citrome, L. (2007). Impact factor? Shmimpact factor!: the journal impact factor, modern day literature searching, and the publication process. *Psychiatry (Edgmont)*, 4 (5), 54–7.

Citrome, L. (2008). Compelling or irrelevant? Using number needed to treat can help decide. *Acta Psychiatr Scand*, 117 (6), 412–19.

Citrome, L. (2009). Quantifying risk: the role of absolute and relative measures in interpreting risk of adverse reactions from product labels of antipsychotic medications. *Curr Drug Saf*, 4 (3), 229–37.

Citrome, L. (2010a). Citability of original research and reviews in journals and their sponsored supplements. *PLoS One*, 5 (3), e9876.

Citrome, L. (2010b). Iloperidone redux: a dissection of the Drug Approval Package for this newly commercialised second-generation antipsychotic. *Int J Clin Pract*, 64 (6), 707–18.

Citrome, L. (2010c). Relative vs. absolute measures of benefit and risk: what's the difference? *Acta Psychiatr Scand*, 121 (2), 94–102

Citrome, L. Call for papers for the International Journal of Clinical Practice. Video. Available at: http://www.youtube.com/watch?v=KBALRk2hjMs. Accessed 2 June 2011.

Citrome, L. and Nasrallah, H. On-label on the table: what the package insert can tell us about the tolerability profile of oral atypical antipsychotics, and what they can't. *Expert Opin Pharmacother*, (in review).

Citrome, L., Moss, S. V., and Graf, C. (2009). How to search and harvest the medical literature: let the citations come to you, and how to proceed when they do. *Int J Clin Pract*, 63 (11), 1565–70.

Clark, J., Gonzalez, J., Mansi, B., *et al.* (2010). Enhancing transparency and efficiency in reporting industry-sponsored clinical research: report from the Medical Publishing Insights and Practices initiative. *Int J Clin Pract*, 64 (8), 1028–33.

ClinicalTrials.gov, a service of the US National Institutes of Health. Available at: www.clinicaltrials.gov. Accessed 2 June 2011.

Cochrane Collaboration. Available at: www.cochrane.org. Accessed 2 June 2011.

Elsevier Embase. Available at: www.embase.com. Accessed 2 June 2011.

Enhancing the Quality and Transparency of Health Research. Available at: http://www.equator-network.org/. Accessed 2 June 2011.

Graf, C., Battisti, W. P., Bridges, D., *et al.* (2009). International Society for Medical Publication Professionals. Research Methods & Reporting. Good publication practice for communicating company sponsored medical research: the GPP2 guidelines. *Brit Med J*, 339, b4330.

International Committee of Medical Journal Editors. Available at: www.icmje.org. Accessed 2 June 2011.

Kraemer, H. C. and Kupfer, D. J. (2006). Size of treatment effects and their importance to clinical research and practice. *Biol Psychiat*, 59 (11), 990–6.

Mathieu, S., Boutron, I., Moher, D., Altman, D. G., and Ravaud, P. (2009). Comparison of registered and published primary outcomes in randomized controlled trials. *J Am Med Assoc*, 302 (9), 977–84.

PubMed.gov, US National Library of Medicine, National Institutes of Health. Available at: http://www.ncbi.nlm.nih.gov/pubmed/. Accessed 2 June 2011.

Schulz, K. F., Altman, D. G., and Moher, D. (2010). CONSORT 2010 statement: updated guidelines for reporting parallel group randomised trials. *J Pharmacol Pharmacother*, 1 (2), 100–7.

Stroup, T. S., McEvoy, J. P., Swartz, M. S., *et al.* (2003). The National Institute of Mental Health Clinical Antipsychotic Trials of Intervention Effectiveness (CATIE) project: schizophrenia trial design and protocol development. *Schizophrenia Bull*, 29 (1), 15–31.

US Food and Drug Administration, Division of Drug Marketing, Advertising, and Communications (DDMAC). Available at: http://www.fda.gov/AboutFDA/CentersOffices/CDER/ucm090142.htm. Accessed 2 June 2011.

The importance of treating cognition in schizophrenia and other severe mental illnesses: background, strategies, and findings to date

Philip D. Harvey and Richard S. E. Keefe

Cognitive impairments have long been known to predict everyday functioning in people with various neuropsychiatric conditions (Heaton and Pendleton, 1981) and schizophrenia is a clear example of that. While there have been multiple reviews and meta-analyses (e.g. Green et al., 2000) of the relationship between cognition and everyday functioning in schizophrenia, recent research has suggested that cognitive deficits may exert their influence on everyday functioning through their relationship with functional capacity (Bowie et al., 2008). Functional capacity refers to the ability to perform the component skills required for everyday functioning, including such things as managing money, making telephone calls, shopping, and traveling (Harvey et al., 2007). It has been found in several studies that cognitive deficits are strongly related to measures of functional capacity, which are in turn related to everyday functioning (see Leifker et al., 2011, for a review). These relationships, presented graphically in Figure 1, suggest that treatment of cognitive impairment may facilitate the chances of improved everyday functioning; moreover, they also suggest that direct improvements in functional capacity, if possible, may also improve everyday outcomes. As can be seen in the figure, of the multiple cognitive domains measured in this study (Bowie et al., 2008), only one had a direct and unmediated influence on the performance-based measures of functional capacity, in this case the UCSD performance-based skills assessment (UPSA; Patterson et al., 2001a) and the Social Skills Performance Assessment (SSPA; Patterson et al., 2001b).

As impairments in everyday functioning are very common and severe in schizophrenia, reducing these deficits is critically important. Impairments in everyday functioning lead to indirect costs of schizophrenia of over $50 billion per year. Those costs are actually greater than the cost of treatment of schizophrenia. For example, the total cost for all antipsychotic treatments administered in the USA in 2010, including to patients with conditions other than schizophrenia, was about $8 billion. Thus, treatments aimed at disability reduction appear to have the potential to lead to marked cost savings to the US economy as a whole.

Cognitive deficits are not produced by the other symptoms of schizophrenia, including hallucinations or disorganization (Keefe et al., 2006a). Clinically stable patients' performance is still considerably impaired, often as much as two or more standard deviations below

Essential CNS Drug Development, ed. A. Kalali, Sheldon Preskorn, J. Kwentus, and Stephen M. Stahl.
Published by Cambridge University Press. © Cambridge University Press 2012.

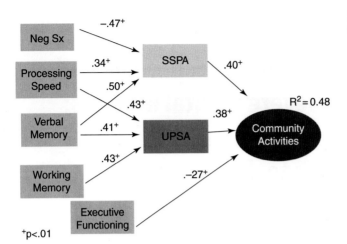

Figure 1. Prediction of community activities.

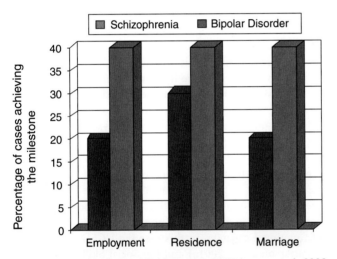

Figure 2. Rates of real-world functional milestones in schizophrenia and bipolar disorder.

From Huxley and Baldessarini, 2007; Leung *et al.*, 2008

expectations based on previous functioning. Thus, treatments that reduce psychosis do not appear to have any notable benefit on cognitive deficits (Keefe *et al.*, 2007); residual disability, despite clinical remission, is quite common (Leung *et al.*, 2008).

A further major issue is the increasingly appreciated fact that patients with bipolar disorder have similar deficits in cognition and everyday functioning, albeit with reduced prevalence of impairment. As noted recently, the rate of disability in patients with bipolar disorder who have recovered symptomatically from at least one mixed or manic episode is about 60% (Huxley and Baldessarini, 2007). As shown in Figure 2, achievement of major lifetime milestones is much more common in bipolar disorder compared to schizophrenia, but is far below that found in the healthy population. Thus, this is another major area of importance for treatment. In a recent meta-analysis of cognition and functioning in bipolar disorder, it has been found that studies that recruited only remitted patients found equivalent cognitive impairments compared to patients with moderate depression symptoms. Thus, although symptoms of depression in bipolar patients may be associated with more severe cognitive impairments, there are substantial residual problems (Wingo *et al.*, 2009), likely requiring treatment, in most patients with bipolar disorder who are clinically stable.

Thus, disability is extraordinarily prevalent in severe mental illness. Treatable components of disability include cognitive deficits and impairments in functional capacity. Although treatment of these two domains of ability does not guarantee success in terms of functional gains, as described below, improving performance in these ability areas is likely a prerequisite for improved everyday functioning.

How to treat cognitive deficits?
Pharmacological interventions
There are several cognitively based conditions where there are currently approved pharmacological treatments. These include attention deficit hyperactivity disorder, where a number of stimulant and non-stimulant treatments are currently approved, and Alzheimer's and Parkinson's dementia, where cholinesterase inhibitors are approved. Thus, it has been documented that aspects of cognition and everyday functioning can be improved through pharmacological means. In addition, pharmacological interventions have recently been approved for the treatment of affective disturbances, including pseudobulbar affect. As a result, pharmacological interventions for cognitive and behavioral syndromes have a history of FDA approval and, in some cases, wide adoption and commercial success.

The US Food and Drug Administration has long adopted a conservative approach for the approval of cognitive enhancing agents. They have expressed a concern that new treatments do not demonstrate their efficacy because they actually impact on other aspects of the illness. Referred to as "pseudospecificity", this refers to the concept that treatment of central aspects of a syndrome cannot receive separate indications. For instance, in the case of Alzheimer's disease, the agency argued that since agitation or functional deficits are central features of Alzheimer's disease, treatments aimed only at these symptoms did not merit a separate indication (Laughren, 2001).

When the original treatments for Alzheimer's disease were evaluated, the agency required evidence not only of cognitive benefit, but also of functional relevance, for the approval of treatments. In the case of Alzheimer's disease, a caregiver rating of the significance of the benefit was routinely used. Given the special circumstances of Alzheimer's disease, which include late-life onset in individuals who have typically achieved at least average levels of life milestones, using a caregiver to corroborate a performance-based assessment seems logical. In the case of severe mental illness, with early onset and symptoms that often interfere with the development and maintenance of normal peer and social relationships, such a requirement might be difficult to fulfill. Further, as noted above, the fact that the existing treatments for schizophrenia do not improve cognition and disability suggests that pseudospecificity arguments probably do not apply to schizophrenia.

An additional issue complicating cognitive enhancing treatment for severe mental illness has been the perceived need to arrive at consensus regarding what aspects of cognition are impaired and should be the target of treatment. Although numerous reviews and meta-analyses had generally defined the range of deficits and their general relationships to everyday functioning, the best strategy for assessment of cognitive functioning as an outcome in a treatment study was not widely agreed upon. As a result, the National Institute

Table 1. MATRICS Consensus Cognitive Battery

Speed of processing:
Category fluency
Brief Assessment of Cognition in Schizophrenia (BACS) – Symbol-Coding
Trail Making A
Attention/vigilance
Continuous Performance Test – Identical Pairs (CPT-IP)
Working memory
Verbal: University of Maryland – Letter-Number Span
Nonverbal: Wechsler Memory Scale (WMS) – III Spatial Span
Verbal learning
Hopkins Verbal Learning Test (HVLT) – Revised
Visual learning
Brief Visuospatial Memory Test (BVMT) – Revised
Reasoning and problem-solving
Neuropsychological Assessment Battery (NAB) – Mazes
Social cognition
Meyer-Solovay-Caruso Emotional Intelligence Test

of Mental Health funded an initiative to define the aspects of cognitive impairment most important to treat in schizophrenia, as well as to comment on research design issues and possible pharmacological strategies to use to treat cognitive deficits. This initiative, named Measurement and Treatment Research to Improve Cognition in Schizophrenia (MATRICS), involved a large segment of the research, pharmacological, and regulatory communities and resulted in several developments. These results are presented in a large number of papers that have been published on this topic (Green *et al.*, 2008; Kern *et al.*, 2008; Neuchterlein *et al.*, 2008). We will largely review the results of the previous studies.

The MATRICS Consensus Cognitive Battery (MCCB)

This cognitive battery, with 10 different tests in six cognitive domains, was developed after a comprehensive consensus development procedure and detailed validation studies. The MCCB has been shown to be highly reliable and easy to complete for people with schizophrenia. A recent study showed that over 99% of 323 people with schizophrenia were able to provide complete data on this assessment (Keefe *et al.*, 2011). Studies of pharmacological and behavioral intervention, to be reviewed below, have shown that the MCCB is sensitive to the effects of these interventions. Table 1 presents the domains and tests that currently constitute the MCCB.

This battery has been co-normed (meaning that normative scores across tests are based on the same healthy sample) and translated and officially validated in several different languages, including several European and Indian languages, several Spanish and Chinese dialects, and

Japanese. This battery has also been examined for its reliability and validity in patients with bipolar disorder, with considerable success (Burdick *et al.*, 2011). Thus, there is an agreed-upon method to examine cognition and changes in cognition with treatment, as developed through an extensive consensus process and endorsed by academic and regulatory agencies.

There are several conceptual aspects of the MCCB that require discussion. The MCCB presumes that cognitive functioning in severe mental illness can be conceptualized by a set of "domains" of functioning. As noted in Table 1, these domains are common neuro-psychological constructs. While the notion that these domains are directly related to the functioning of discrete regions of the brain has been discarded, there is still some debate as to whether these domains have validity in terms of specific relationships with different elements of everyday functioning, such as social vs. vocational functioning. A final issue for consideration is whether these domains require more than a single task for their definition. Many of the MCCB domains are defined by a single assessment procedure. Thus, they are really not scientific constructs defined by the convergence of multiple related tests, but rather single representative tests within different domains. This situation is difficult to avoid, as more tests per domain would result in a longer battery. The trade-off in this situation is clearly practicality vs. scientific purity, which was discussed extensively during the development of the battery. As there have been published critiques of the MCCB arguing that it is too long (Silverstein *et al.*, 2010), the addition of more tests to establish domain specificity may not be pragmatic.

The dimensionality of the MCCB is, in a sense, a minor argument given the fact that the recommendation of the developers was that an average or "composite" score, weighting all domains equally, should be the outcomes measure used for treatment studies (Neuchterlein *et al.*, 2008). This choice is well supported by previous findings suggesting that abbreviated assessments or subsets of longer batteries are very well correlated with longer batteries (Harvey *et al.*, 2009; Keefe *et al.*, 2004, 2006b). Further, in comparative studies, composite scores, from longer and shorter assessment batteries, have been found to have greater test-retest stability and considerably higher correlations with functional outcomes measures than individual tests or cognitive domains (e.g. Leifker *et al.*, 2010).

Cognitive enhancement research design

In addition to the consensus outcomes assessment battery, an additional product of the MATRICS process was a suggested research design to demonstrate cognitive enhancement (Buchanan *et al.*, 2005, 2010). This is also well described in the original and revised papers, but there are several important features worth noting here. Patients who enter the trial should be generally clinically stable with only moderate to less severe symptoms. Their treatment should be stable on one or more antipsychotic medications for an extended period of time and the treatment trial should be long enough (6 months, albeit this is debatable) to suggest that the effects are at least minimally durable. No medications that affect cognitive functioning (such as anticholinergics or antihistamines) should be received during the treatment trial. These requirements are in place to ensure that the specific cognitive enhancement interventions are responsible for any cognitive changes that are detected and that these changes are not due to improvements in symptoms, changes in the underlying treatments, or random variance in symptoms over time.

Part of the reason for these suggestions was the concern expressed by regulators that treatments that might be approved for an indication of cognitive enhancement are only indirectly effective. Theoretically at least, improvements in psychosis might lead to improvements in performance-based assessments. Thus, the changes in cognitive performance would not be due to a change in the underlying cognitive deficit, but rather in the general levels of symptoms on the part of the patient. As reviewed above, this concern in schizophrenia seems minimally important, in that psychosis does not affect the level of measured cognitive symptoms. However, in mood-disordered populations, including major depression and bipolar disorder, there is some contribution of symptomatic severity, particularly the severity of depression, to cognitive deficits (Wingo *et al.*, 2009). Thus, treatments that specifically enhance cognition would be seen as candidates for approval specifically as cognitive enhancers, while treatments that improved cognition in the context of also reducing global symptom severity would be regulated differently.

Augmentation therapy as a treatment strategy

As in many other conditions, the presumption of the core research design is that cognitive enhancing agents will be added to ongoing primary treatments for the mental illness in question. This strategy is commonly used in many other disease areas such as cardiac conditions and cancer, where multiple treatments are commonly combined in order to provide optimal disease management. As noted above, stable illness management treatment will be delivered and augmentation therapy would be delivered, at first in clinical trials and then later in clinical treatment of schizophrenia.

Validation of co-primary measures

As noted above, FDA representatives have requested that studies of cognitive enhancement also demonstrate clinical applicability by proving that changes in the primary outcomes have some type of functional relevance. These functionally relevant outcome measures have several possible forms, including measures of community functioning, such as obtaining a job, renting one's own apartment, or getting engaged or married. These seem to be implausible outcomes in short-term trials, even of 6 months duration. Finally, certain classes of observers can determine that a patient appears more capable, in that they either perform more functionally important acts, achieve more milestones, or that their general level of competence appears to improve whether or not their life circumstances change (Harvey *et al.*, 2011b).

All of these outcome measures are intrinsically valid, but they are differentially affected by extraneous factors that have nothing to do with the success of treatments. For example, real-world milestones are often difficult to achieve rapidly in the population as a whole, because of circumstances such as personnel department delays associated with being hired at a new job, the need to save money to pay a security deposit to live independently in a new apartment, and the fact that long-term relationships such as marriage need to develop over the long term. As a result, achievement of these milestones would not be a sensible outcome measure even in a study of healthy people; this expectation is even more unrealistic in those with severe and persistent mental illnesses. Observer reports of functionality are potentially limited by several factors. Limited contact with the patient, reduced opportunity to observe the behaviors of importance, and the observer's own response biases, illnesses, and ability to report accurately in general are all potential factors reducing the validity of observer report. The availability of informants may also be an issue. Some people with schizophrenia report that they have no available informants (Patterson *et al.*, 1996)

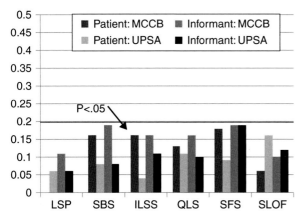

Figure 3. Correlations between ability scores and reported functioning: friend/relative informant.

Note. LSP: Life Skills Profile; SBS: Social Behavior Schedule; ILSS: Independent Living Skills Survey; QLS: Heinrichs Carpenter Quality of Life Scale; SFS: Social Functioning Scale; SLOF: Specific Levels of Functioning.

and at the same time several large studies involving informant reports have been completed recently (Harvey *et al.*, 2011a,b). There are some suggestions that not all informants give equally valid reports (Sabbag *et al.*, in press) and the search to find any informant who is willing to participate may lead to reduced validity.

It is tempting to ask people with severe mental illness how they are functioning, but there are multiple pitfalls with this approach. Not even healthy individuals are able to provide accurate self-assessments of their functional abilities (Dunning and Story, 1991). People with schizophrenia regularly provide essentially random reports of their functioning (Bowie *et al.*, 2007; McKibbin *et al.*, 2004); the correlations between self-reports, objectively achieved milestones, and the validated reports of observers approach zero.

As documented in a recent paper (Sabbag *et al.*, in press), self-reports and the reports of friend or relative informants were very poorly correlated with patients' performance on ability-based assessments. In this study, high-contact clinicians or friends or relatives provided reports of patients' everyday functioning on six different functional rating scales, while patients provided self-reports of their functioning. These scales measured daily activities, social functioning, and vocational readiness. Patients also performed one of the standard functional capacity measures, the UPSA-B, and the MCCB as a cognitive measure, with the informants unaware of those scores.

As shown in Figure 3, the two ability-based measures in the patients were uncorrelated with friend or relative informant reports and self-reports. In contrast, as shown in Figure 4, even in a smaller sample the correlations of the ability-based measures with the clinician-informant reports were considerably higher and consistent with our previous studies examining the correlation between clinician reports and patient performance.

The primary solution proposed for biased and inaccurate reports provided by inform-ants has been to measure abilities directly. As noted above, the functional capacity assess-ment strategy has been found to have considerable validity. In one of the later steps of the MATRICS project, a study validating different strategies for co-primary measures was conducted (Green *et al.*, 2011). This study examined self-reported cognitive and functional

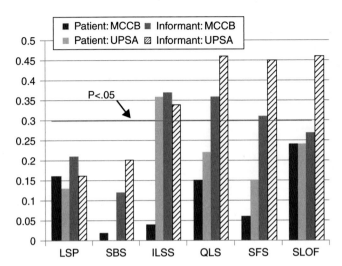

Figure 4. Correlations between ability scores and reported functioning: clinician informant.

Note. LSP: Life Skills Profile; SBS: Social Behavior Schedule; ILSS: Independent Living Skills Survey; QLS: Heinrichs Carpenter Quality of Life Scale; SFS: Social Functioning Scale; SLOF: Specific Levels of Functioning.

abilities and several different performance-based measures of functional capacity for their temporal stability and convergent validity with cognitive performance indexed with the MCCB. It was found that performance-based measures were uniformly more strongly correlated with the MCCB than self-reported cognitive functioning, with the UPSA performing best of the performance-based measures. Self-reported cognitive functioning was only weakly related to the MCCB. Abbreviated versions of the performance-based functional capacity measures were also examined and the results of the study revealed that abbreviated measures (e.g. two of five UPSA subtests) performed quite well compared to longer versions of the assessments.

The conclusions of these studies were that co-primary measures were valid and practical and actually took considerably less time to administer than the MCCB, with no more missing data than the primary assessments. While there are no definitive data to date regarding the differential sensitivity of primary (MCCB) and co-primary (UPSA) outcome measures to treatments, pharmacological or behavioral, this is an important research area for the immediate future.

Pharmacological enhancement results

As reviewed recently (Harvey, 2009), the results of pharmacological cognitive enhancement studies have generally been negative, with a few recent positive results that need confirmation. Many of the earlier studies were severely underpowered, used less comprehensive assessment than the MCCB, and a relatively small proportion of the completed studies employed co-primary outcome measures. However, negative findings have been common across studies.

While a detailed review is outside the scope of this chapter, other comprehensive reviews have suggested that multiple mechanisms have not met with considerable success. See Table 2

Table 2. Compounds and mechanisms of action in cognitive enhancement studies

General pharmacological domain	Compounds	Mechanisms of action
Cholinergic		
Muscarinic	Donepezil	Acetylcholinesterase inhibition
	Galantamine	Acetylcholinesterase inhibition
	Rivastigmine	Acetylcholinesterase inhibition
Nicotinic	DMX-B	Alpha-7 partial agonist
	AZD3480	Alpha-4-beta-2 agonist
Glutamatergic	Glycine	NMDA co-transmitter
	d-cyloserine	NMDA glycine site partial agonist
	CX-516	AMPA-Kine (allosteric modulator)
	Lamotrigine	Glutamate release regulation
Noradrenergic	Guanfacine	Alpha-2 agonist
	Atomoxetine	Transport inhibitor
γ-Aminobutyric acid	Flumazenil	$GABA_A$ antagonist
	MK-0777	$GABA_{A23}$ antagonist
Serotonergic	Tandospirone	$5\text{-}HT_{1a}$ partial agonist
	Buspirone	$5\text{-}HT_{1a}$ partial agonist
Dopaminergic	Tolcapone	COMT inhibitor
Stimulant	Amphetamine	Agonist and transport inhibitor
Alertness agents	Modafinil	Unknown

for a partial list of previous mechanisms attempted. We have discussed the possible reasons for failure of these trials previously (Harvey, 2009; Harvey and McClure, 2006). It is noteworthy that many of the trials to date have included patients who are older, largely male, and have long durations of illness. While only empirical studies can sufficiently address the question of which patients are the most responsive to cognitive enhancement treatment, the characteristics of patients in most previous studies may not be ideal for treatments that may need to take advantage of neural mechanisms of neuroplasticity to be fully effective. Another possibility is that pharmacological treatment alone may not be sufficient to change performance on cognitive performance measures. It may be the case that some sort of supportive or evocative additional intervention may be required in order to detect changes. As described in detail in the sections below on cognitive remediation, this idea has already received considerable support.

Nonpharmacological interventions

Cognitive remediation interventions have begun to be broadly studied for use with people with severe mental illness. Recent developments in the delivery of these interventions (see McGurk *et al.*, 2007b, for a review) have led to substantial increases in the extent to which they improve performance on cognitive tests and, more importantly, improve everyday functioning in multiple domains. These interventions have several common features that separate them from earlier interventions. In addition, the methodology for delivering and dosing these programs has improved. Finally, understanding the concurrent support systems, other functional enhancing interventions, and spacing of the delivery of cognitive enhancement sessions has helped to determine what constitutes an effective intervention.

Strategies. There are two broad classes of cognitive remediation intervention strategies. These include strategies that are "top-down" models, where the interventions are broadly based and target motor processes. Examples of such strategies could include training on problem-solving procedures (McGurk *et al.*, 2005), where the problem-solving procedures require the deployment of multiple component tests such as perception, attention, concentration, working memory, and episodic memory in order to succeed on the test. This strategy is based on both the notion of efficiency of intervention delivery (i.e. it is best to train everything at once) and on the notion that global cognitive abilities are the most proximal determinant of everyday outcomes.

The second strategy, also employed with success to date, is the bottom-up strategy. Such a strategy is based on the concept that there are certain brain regions that have been found to be uniformly impaired in various neuropsychiatric conditions and that increasing the functioning of that brain region will have a generalized benefit on a multitude of distal cognitive abilities that rely in part on the functioning of that brain region (Fisher *et al.*, 2009). An example of this procedure would be extensively training individuals on elements of auditory information processing, with the stimuli initially being non-verbal and the training demands increasing in complexity over time.

Dosing

Scheduling. Dosing cognitive remediation requires careful consideration (Medalia *et al.*, 2009). It is a central tenet of experimental psychology that massed practice provides more durable learning than spaced practice, but the definition of massed and spaced may be somewhat flexible, particularly in populations with cognitive compromise. Most critical is the question of what to do with patient participants who miss sessions and need to make them up. The core characteristics of disorganization in schizophrenia essentially guarantee that outpatients with the condition will miss some training sessions. One strategy commonly applied is that of making up sessions on a structured basis, with participants allowed to perform two training sessions on days when they arrive for training and only terminating patients from research studies if they miss more than two consecutive weeks of training (Keefe *et al.*, 2011).

Number of sessions. The actual required dose for benefit is still a work in progress. In studies demonstrating the efficacy of top-down interventions, studies have aimed for completion of 2–3 training sessions per week over 12 weeks (actual mean completion = 19.6 hours) (McGurk *et al.*, 2005). When a similar study, with the same cognitive remediation strategy, was conducted with chronically institutionalized inpatients, these participants completed an average of 20 sessions (Lindenmayer *et al.*, 2008). A study examining the efficacy of bottom-up interventions aimed for 1 hour sessions, 5 days per week for 10 weeks (actual mean completion = 47.9 hours) (Fisher *et al.*, 2009). Thus, there is considerable variability in the dosing associated with successful cognitive remediation treatment. At this time, it is not possible to offer a definitive answer as to the minimum number of sessions required for an effect, but the findings of the McGurk and Lindenmayer *et al.* studies above suggest that functionally relevant benefits can be obtained after about 20 sessions, at least with top-down interventions.

Magnitude of effect. Cognitive remediation has been remarkably successful in improving cognitive performance in people with schizophrenia. In certain studies with co-administered therapies, there have been substantial functional benefits as well.

Cognitive change. Cognitive deficits in schizophrenia are substantial, so the question arises as to how much improvement would be meaningful, or even detectable, to observers. It is, therefore, difficult to index how much improvement would lead to functional gains. This question is not possible to answer without concurrent functional assessments, but there are some studies that suggest substantial cognitive gains. These results will be presented in terms of effect sizes, which give an unbiased estimate of the magnitude of change that operates independently of the sample size.

The classic definitions of effect sizes define changes in terms of the proportion of a standard deviation from baseline. Small effects are defined as 0.2 SD, medium effects are defined as 0.5 SD, and large effects are defined as 0.8 SD. Previous research has indicated that observers with no training or instructions can detect medium effect sizes for differences between two groups. Thus, medium effect sizes approach those that would be considered functionally meaningful. An influential meta-analysis of contemporary cognitive remediation studies suggested that the average effect size for cognitive remediation interventions was .41 for cognition and .36 for everyday functioning (McGurk *et al.*, 2007b). The conclusion from this review was that the benefit of cognitive remediation was meaningful, but variable across studies.

Since that review, there have been several additional studies published. A more recent meta-analysis (Wykes *et al.*, 2011) confirmed that the effect of cognitive remediation has a mean effect of 0.45 SD and a 95% confidence interval of .31 to .59, overlapping the classic metric of a medium effect. In sum, there is significant evidence that cognitive remediation regularly produces substantial cognitive benefits.

Functional outcomes. Functional outcomes are the ultimate goal of treatment of cognitive impairments. Most studies of cognitive remediation have measured these outcomes, as noted above. For example, in the McGurk *et al.* (2007a) 36-month study, work outcomes were substantially better in the intervention group compared to the control group. For number of hours worked over 3 years, the intervention group worked 897% more hours. They also earned 1000% more money. So, an average of 19 hours of cognitive remediation led to a 10-fold increase in earning and a 9-fold increase in hours worked. In the Fisher *et al.* study (2010), functional gains were also realized. In a larger sample, they were able to prove that cognitive gains in remediation were also associated with clinician-rated improvements in functioning. As a result, cognitive improvements are found to lead to functional gains, validating the notion that cognitive enhancement leads to functional improvements in people with schizophrenia.

Concurrent treatments. A recent meta-analysis addressed several of the issues associated with cognitive remediation as a treatment strategy. These include dosing of treatment and other indices associated with methodological rigor. It was found that clinical stability predicted greater benefit from enhancement therapy, as did the provision of concurrent psychosocial interventions (Wykes *et al.*, 2011). Strategy, dose, and in-person versus computer treatment did not affect efficacy, but the more structured the concurrent psychosocial intervention, the greater the treatment response. So, even cognitive remediation treatments with demonstrated efficacy produce better results when combined with psychosocial interventions.

Cognitive remediation as a platform for pharmacological studies

It is possible that many of the experimental pharmacological interventions will be of only minimal benefit when patients are evaluated in the context of their habitual low level of cognitive stimulation. Part of the explanation for why clinical trials testing the efficacy of cognitive-enhancing medications have so far been largely unsuccessful may be that patients in these trials are not provided with substantive opportunity to utilize the cognitive benefit that they may have acquired during the drug treatment study. Thus, analogous to the need for physical exercise in an individual who takes steroids to increase muscle mass, schizophrenia patients in pharmacological intervention trials may require systematic cognitive training to "exercise" any newfound cognitive potential that they may have acquired from drug treatment (Keefe *et al.*, 2010).

Cognitive remediation may provide an excellent platform for enriching the cognitive environment of patients engaged in pharmacological trials to improve cognition. As noted above, cognitive remediation produces medium to large effect size improvements in cognitive performance and, when combined with psychiatric rehabilitation, also improves functional outcomes (Lindenmayer *et al.*, 2008; McGurk *et al.*, 2007b; Wykes *et al.*, 2011). Patients find these programs to be enjoyable and engaging, and they have been linked with increases in participant self-esteem. Ongoing treatment with cognitive remediation may thus provide schizophrenia patients with the necessary cognitive enrichment and motivation to demonstrate the true potential of effective cognitive enhancement with pharmacological intervention. Recent work suggests that these methods are feasible in clinical trials even at sites without cognitive remediation experience (Keefe *et al.*, 2011).

Conclusions

Cognitive impairment is a functionally relevant, albeit challenging treatment target. In contrast to symptoms of neuropsychiatric conditions, behavioral interventions have reliably produced better treatment effects than pharmacological interventions. However, combined therapies may result in better outcomes, with the meta-analytic finding that cognitive remediation reliably produces better effects when combined with psychosocial interventions suggesting combination therapies as the way forward.

Cognitive impairment is a critical treatment goal and the promise of cognitive treatment is moving forward. Thus far, pharmacological treatments are lagging behind the results of cognitive remediation interventions. It is possible that combined interventions may be better even in the area of enhancing performance on cognitive tests and this may improve outcomes for pharmacological treatments. No pharmacological studies have required psychosocial interventions to occur concurrently to pharmacological interventions. As some studies have suggested that motivational deficits deleteriously impact improvements in treatment trials, it may be the case that psychosocial interventions can overcome some of these barriers to treatment even in pharmacological studies.

References

Bowie, C. R., Twamley, E. W., Anderson, H., et al. (2007). Self-assessment of functional status in schizophrenia. *J Psychiatr Res*, 41, 1012–18.

Bowie, C. R., Leung, W. W., Reichenberg, A., et al. (2008). Predicting schizophrenia patients' real world behavior with specific neuropsychological and functional capacity measures. *Biol Psychiat*, 63, 505–11.

Buchanan, R. W., Davis, M., Goff, D., et al. (2005). A summary of the FDA-NIMH-MATRICS workshop on clinical trial design for neurocognitive drugs for schizophrenia. *Schizophrenia Bull*, 31, 5–19.

Buchanan, R. W., Keefe, R. S. E., Umbricht, D., et al. (2010). The FDA-NIMH-MATRICS guidelines for clinical trial design of cognitive-enhancing drugs: What do we know 5 years later? *Schizophrenia Bull*, [epub ahead of print].

Burdick, K. E., Goldberg, T. E., Cornblatt, B. A., et al. (2011). The MATRICS Consensus Cognitive Battery in Patients with Bipolar I Disorder. *Neuropsychopharmacology*, 36, 1587–92.

Dunning, D. and Story, A. L. (1991). Depression, realism, and the overconfidence effect: are the sadder wiser when predicting future actions and events? *J Person Soc Psychol*, 61, 521–32.

Fisher, M., Holland, C., Merzenich, M. M., and Vinogradov, S. (2009). Using neuroplasticity-based auditory training to improve verbal memory in schizophrenia. *Am J Psychiat*, 166, 805–11.

Fisher, M., Holland, C., Subramaniam, K., and Vinogradov, S. (2010). Neuroplasticity-based cognitive training in schizophrenia: An interim report on the effects 6 months later. *Schizophrenia Bull*, 36, 869–79.

Green, M. F., Kern, R. S., Braff, D. L., and Mintz, J. (2000). Neurocognitive deficits and functional outcome in schizophrenia: Are we measuring the "right stuff"? *Schizophrenia Bull*, 26, 119–36.

Green, M. F., Nuechterlein, K. H., and Kern, R. S. (2008). Functional co-primary measures for clinical trials in schizophrenia: results from the MATRICS Psychometric and Standardization Study. *Am J Psychiat*, 165, 221–8.

Green, M. F., Schooler, N. R., Kern, R. D., et al. (2011). Evaluation of functionally-meaningful measures for clinical trials of cognition enhancement in schizophrenia. *Am J Psychiat*, 168, 400–7.

Harvey, P. D. (2009). Pharmacological cognitive enhancement in schizophrenia. *Neuropsychol Rev*, 19, 324–35.

Harvey, P. D. and McClure, M. M. (2006). Pharmacological approaches to the management of cognitive dysfunction in schizophrenia. *Drugs*, 66, 1465–73.

Harvey, P. D., Velligan, D. I., and Bellack, A. S. (2007). Performance-based measures of functional skills: usefulness in clinical treatment studies. *Schizophrenia Bull*, 33, 1138–48.

Harvey, P. D., Keefe, R. S. E., Patterson, T. L., Heaton, R. K., and Bowie, C. R. (2009). Abbreviated neuropsychological assessments in schizophrenia: Association with different outcomes measures. *J Clin Exp Neuropsychol*, 31, 462–71.

Harvey, P. D., Ogasa, M., Cucchiaro, J., Loebel, A., and Keefe, R. S. E. (2011a). Performance and interview-based assessments of cognitive change in a randomized, double-blind comparison of lurasidone vs. ziprasidone. *Schizophr Res*, 127, 188–94.

Harvey, P. D., Raykov, T., Twamley, E. M., et al. (2011b). In press. Validating the measurement of real-world functional outcome: Phase I results of the VALERO study. *Am J Psychiat*.

Heaton, R. K. and Pendleton, M. G. (1981). Use of neuropsychological tests to predict patients' everyday functioning. *J Con Consult Psychol*, 49, 807–21.

Huxley, N. and Baldessarini, R. J. (2007). Disability and its treatment in bipolar disorder patients. *Bipolar Disorder*, 9, 183–96.

Keefe, R. S., Goldberg, T. E., Harvey, P. D., et al. (2004). The Brief Assessment of Cognition in Schizophrenia: reliability, sensitivity, and comparison with a standard neurocognitive battery. *Schizophr Res*, 68, 283–97.

Keefe, R. S. E., Bilder, R. M., Harvey, P. D., et al. (2006a). Baseline neurocognitive deficits in the CATIE schizophrenia trial. *Neuropsychopharmacology*, 31, 2033–46.

Keefe, R. S. E., Poe, M., Walker, T. M., Kang, J. W., and Harvey, P. D. (2006b). The schizophrenia cognition rating scale: An interview-based assessment and its relationship to cognition, real-world functioning, and functional capacity. *Am J Psychiat*, 163, 426–32.

Keefe, R. S. E., Bilder, R. M., Davis, S. M., et al. (2007). Neurocognitive effects of antipsychotic medications in patients with chronic schizophrenia in the CATIE trial. *Arch Gen Psychiat*, 64, 633–47.

Keefe, R. S. E., Vinogradov, S., Medalia, A., et al. (2010). Report from the Working Group Conference on multi-site trial design for cognitive remediation in schizophrenia. *Schizophrenia Bull*, doi: 10.1093/schbul/sub010.

Keefe, R. S. E., Fox, K. H., Harvey, P. D., et al. (2011). Characteristics of the MATRICS Consensus Cognitive Battery in a 29-site antipsychotic schizophrenia clinical trial. *Schizophr Res*, 125, 161–8.

Kern, R. S., Nuechterlein, K. H., Green, M. F., et al. (2008). The MATRICS Consensus Cognitive Battery: Part 2. Co-norming and standardization. *Am J Psychiat*, 165, 214–20.

Laughren, T. (2001). A regulatory perspective on psychiatric syndromes in Alzheimer's disease. *Am J Geriatr Psychiat*, 9, 340–5.

Leifker, F. R., Patterson, T. L., Bowie, C. R., Mausbach, B. T., and Harvey, P. D. (2010). Psychometric properties of performance-based measurements of functional capacity: test-retest reliability, practice effects, and potential sensitivity to change. *Schizophr Res*, 119, 246–52.

Leifker, F. R., Patterson, T. L., Heaton, R. K., and Harvey, P. D. (2011). Validating measures of real-world outcome: the results of the VALERO Expert Survey and RAND Panel. *Schizophrenia Bull*, 37, 334–43.

Leung, W. W., Bowie, C. R., and Harvey, P. D. (2008). Functional implications of neuropsychological normality and symptom remission in older outpatients diagnosed with schizophrenia: a cross-sectional study. *J Int Neuropsychol Soc*, 14, 479–88.

Lindenmayer, J. P., McGurk, S. R., Mueser, K. T., et al. (2008). A randomized controlled trial of cognitive remediation among inpatients with persistent mental illness. *Psychiatric Serv*, 59, 241–7.

McClure, M. M., Bowie, C. R., Patterson, T. L., et al. (2007). Correlations of functional capacity and neuropsychological performance in older patients with schizophrenia: evidence for specificity of relationships? *Schizophr Res*, 89, 330–8.

McGurk, S. R., Mueser, K. T., and Pascaris, A. (2005). Cognitive training and supported employment for persons with severe mental illness: one-year results from a randomized controlled trial. *Schizophrenia Bull*, 31, 898–909.

McGurk, S. R., Mueser, K. T., Feldman, K., Wolfe, R., and Pascaris, A. (2007a). Cognitive training for supported employment: 2–3 year outcomes of a randomized controlled trial. *Am J Psychiat*, 164, 437–41.

McGurk, S. R., Twamley, E. W., Sitzer, D. I., McHugo, G. J., and Mueser, K. T. (2007b). A meta-analysis of cognitive remediation in schizophrenia. *Am J Psychiat*, 164, 1791–802.

McKibbin, C., Patterson, T. L., and Jeste, D. V. (2004). Assessing disability in older patients with schizophrenia: results from the WHODAS-II. *J Nerv Ment Dis*, 192, 405–13.

Medalia, A., Revheim, N., and Herlands, T. (2009). *Cognitive Remediation for Psychological Disorders, Therapist Guide*. New York: Oxford University Press.

Neuchterlein, K. H., Green, M. F., Kern, R. S., et al. (2008). The MATRICS Consensus Cognitive Battery: Part 1. Test selection, reliability, and validity. *Am J Psychiat*, 165, 203–13.

Patterson, T. L., Semple, S. J., Shaw, W. S., Grant, I., and Jeste, D. V. (1996). Researching the caregiver: family members who care for older psychotic patients. *Psychiatr Ann*, 26, 772–84.

Patterson, T. L., Goldman, S., McKibbin, C. L., Hughs, T., and Jeste, D. V. (2001a). UCSD performance-based skills assessment: development of a new measure of everyday functioning for severely mentally ill adults. *Schizophrenia Bull*, 27, 235–45.

Patterson, T. L., Moscona, S., McKibbin, C. L., Davidson, K., and Jeste, D. V. (2001b). Social skills performance assessment among older patients with schizophrenia. *Schizophr Res*, 48, 351–60.

Sabbag, S., Twamley, E. W., Vella, L., Heaton, R. K., Patterson, T. L., and Harvey, P. D. (2011). Assessing everyday functioning in schizophrenia: Not all informants seem equally informative. *Schizophr Res*, 131, 250–5.

Silverstein, S. M., Jaeger, J., Donovan-Lepore, A. M., *et al.* (2010). A comparative study of the MATRICS and IntegNeuro cognitive assessment batteries. *J Clin Exp Neuropsychol*, 32 (9), 937–52.

Wingo, A., Harvey, P. D., and Baldessarini, R. J. (2009). Neurocognitive impairment in bipolar disorder patients: functional implications. *Bipolar Disord*, 11, 113–25.

Wykes, T., Huddy, V., Cellard, C., McGurk, S. R., and Czobor, P. (2011). A meta-analysis of cognitive remediation for schizophrenia: methodology and effect sizes. *Am J Psychiat*, 168 (5), 472–85.

Chapter 3

Leveraging disruptive technologies to drive innovation in CNS clinical drug development

Penny Randall, Judith Dunn, and Amir Kalali

Disruptive technologies and drug development

Over the last decade, sizeable investments have been made by both private and public entities in various technologies to improve health outcomes and to drive down the cost of managing illness. This chapter will review recent technological advancements that are currently being applied in clinical medicine and explore how the pharmaceutical industry might integrate these technologies to drive innovation through the drug development process as well as product development.

The best example of where investments in technology and infrastructure are beginning to have a real impact on delivery of clinical care is the area of wireless health or mobile health, where a large and varied ecosystem has emerged to support wireless solutions in healthcare delivery (Figure 1). This ecosystem, including sensors, infrastructure, devices, and applications, creates considerable opportunities for value creation in general for clinical medicine and drug development and specifically for CNS drug development.

The wireless ecosystem is already beginning to reshape the general practice of clinical medicine and providing evidence of superior outcomes compared to the standard of care. As just one example, the largest reported study of clinical outcomes in congestive heart failure ($n = 194\,006$), the ALTITUDE study, showed the immense value of remote monitoring. Patients with implantable devices (implantable cardioverter-defibrillators and cardiac resynchronization therapy devices) with remote monitoring demonstrated significantly improved 1- and 5-year survival rates compared to patients with implantable devices that were not connected, and thus received follow-up only in clinic visits (Saxon and Gilliam, 2010).

Wireless health technology

A variety of wireless sensors are now available that allow for the automatic collection of physiological data that are communicated via a gateway, such as a smart phone, to remote systems, where the data can be used by healthcare professionals to manage the care. The types of data that can now be captured by wireless sensors and remotely monitored are quite broad and include body temperature, blood pressure, respiratory rate, heart rate and heart rate variability analysis, ECG tracings, glucose levels, ultrasound images, respiratory spirometry, fluid volume levels, oxygen saturation, activity levels, single-channel EEG data, and even polysomnography data (Figures 1 and 2).

Essential CNS Drug Development, ed. A. Kalali, Sheldon Preskorn, J. Kwentus, and Stephen M. Stahl. Published by Cambridge University Press. © Cambridge University Press 2012.

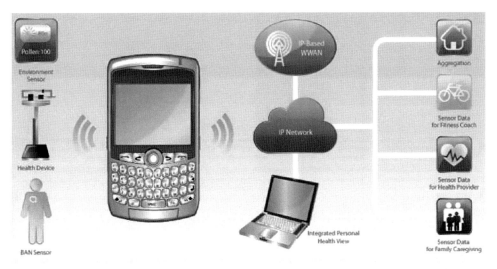

Figure 1. Emerging ecosystem of connectivity in healthcare *(Source: West Wireless Health Institute)*. Wireless capabilities are being built into dedicated devices for remote care and monitoring. This emerging wireless ecosystem presents tremendous opportunities for use in clinical research.

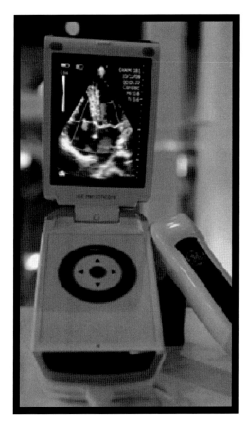

Figure 2. GE V-scan device. GE and other medical equipment manufacturers have developed small mobile ultrasound equipment. From these relatively inexpensive units, images can be wirelessly relayed from the patient to healthcare providers, limiting the use of more expensive, hospital-based diagnostic testing to a smaller subset of patients.

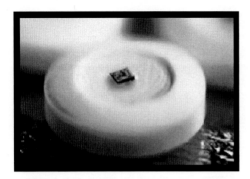

Figure 3. Novartis's antihypertensive Diovan tablet (valsartan) embedded with an ingestible wireless sensor. Source: *Financial Times*, September 21, 2009.

Wireless technology and clinical drug development

Pharmaceutical companies have already begun to apply wireless sensor technologies to clinical trials and product development. The two cases that follow illustrate different ways in which companies have used this disruptive technology. In the first case, Novartis studied combining wireless sensor technology with its top-selling antihypertensive to monitor compliance of the medication. The second case illustrates how a large, global pharmaceutical company created value by amplifying signal detection to accelerate clinical trials.

Novartis and Proteus Biomedical have collaborated and have released impressive findings from a small study, which looked at patient compliance with Novartis's branded antihypertensive, Diovan (valsartan) combined with Proteus Biomedical's wireless sensor. Proteus Biomedical has developed an ingestible wireless sensor that is paired with an external patch. The patch is affixed to the patient's body. The ingestible sensor is small, only 1 mm square and 200 μm thick, and is embedded into the Diovan tablet. When swallowed, the sensor transmits a signal to the patch to indicate patient compliance. In addition to tracking medication compliance, the patch captures and communicates a continuous stream of vital sign data to remote data systems via a smart phone gateway. Healthcare professionals have access to the information about medication compliance as well as real-time drug tolerability data.

Novartis reported that patient compliance improved from 30% for standard Diovan tablets to 80% for the sensor-embedded version. The gains in compliance occurred because subjects who received the sensor-embedded Diovan and failed to take the antihypertensive daily were sent a reminder text message to their smart phone (Jack, 2009).

Given the impressive results from the Diovan trial, Novartis and Proteus Biomedical are testing the technology in schizophrenia to evaluate whether the technology will have a similar impact on medication compliance in this clinically challenging disorder.

Proteus Biomedical has positioned its technology platform (ingestible sensor and smart patch that collects and analyzes physiological data) as not only a tool to improve medication compliance, but a system that can offer a real-world, improved therapeutic effect, by monitoring compliance and managing individual tolerability to the drug.

In the second example, a large pharmaceutical company signed a licensing agreement this year with NeuroVigil, a San Diego-based biomedical company. NeuroVigil developed a wireless EEG sensor supported by a proprietary algorithm coded into software to capture and to analyze subtle abnormalities in brain activity. The pharmaceutical company plans to use this sensor in many of its outpatient clinical trials to identify toxicities, even before the onset of adverse events or before cognitive symptoms are detected clinically. By integrating this wireless sensor into various protocols, Roche expects to acquire high-quality data about drug toxicity in a low-cost setting (i.e. at the subject's home) to better inform dose-finding and go/no go decisions. Roche also intends to establish a comprehensive library of sensor-derived EEG data for molecules, which will be used to predict toxicities of new molecules with similar structures to those archived in the library.

This platform and other emerging technologies illustrate ways for the industry to successfully emerge from its current turmoil related to the revenue shortfalls stemming from the loss of patent protection on many of its blockbuster drugs.

These two examples point to some of the benefits that can be derived from the integration of wireless technology in clinical research, including improved study drug compliance, better information about drug tolerability and safety, and ultimately higher-quality research.

New business models will emerge that focus on developing products that achieve real and measurable improvements in health outcomes (versus the historic focus on introducing new drugs of only marginal benefit, or worse, me-too drugs). The industry has its best chance to regain its competitive footing through this product transformation (Cutler, 2007).

Strategic opportunities for CNS drug developers

Fundamentally, wireless technology allows the capture and analysis of real-time, continuous physiological data at relatively low cost and allows for a range of benefits in drug development. Broadly, the application of wireless technology in clinical research could improve services and generate value through:

(1) enhanced ability to detect safety and efficacy signals;
(2) development of new physiological outcomes measures or biomarkers;
(3) improved study medication compliance and verification of compliance;
(4) acceleration of clinical trials (as a second-order effect), due to enhanced signal detection;
(5) reduction of trial costs through remote trial platforms (i.e. direct-to-participant trials).

Benefits

Wireless sensor technology can be leveraged to provide greater clarity on drug safety, tolerability, and efficacy. Having more robust data is transformative: drugs can be developed faster and more cheaply. Uncertainty about a drug's optimal dose range is reduced. There is greater understanding about the compound's safety profile, and new ways to measure clinical efficacy are possible. Finally, better information will enable drug developers to make more informed decisions about investments in their pipelines, namely, when to move forward with a compound versus when to end its development.

Signal detection

The biomedical company Corventis, for example, has developed a sensor called PiiX that captures the following data continuously: temperature, heart rate, blood pressure, fluid volume, activity level, ECG data, and heart rate variability. The sensor was developed to detect early signs (sub-clinical) of cardiac decompensation in congestive heart failure (CHF) patients.

Across all phases of CNS clinical research, the integration of this type of sensor could greatly enhance knowledge about the safety, tolerability, and, depending on the indication, efficacy of the compound in development. In early Phase II/III trials, the sensor can provide robust data about real-time tolerability following dosing, and facilitate dose-finding. In some indications, the sensor can be used to provide data supportive of an efficacy claim such as in the development of an antihypertensive or a drug to treat CHF. In trials that evaluate treatments for renal insufficiency, real-time information about fluid volume status would be invaluable.

Biomarkers

The large variety of wireless sensor data available offers the opportunity to reconsider how safety and efficacy are evaluated. The use of sensor data can lead to the development of a new set of vital signs or biomarkers for trials based on the specific challenges associated with an indication. The NeuroVigil sensor, for example, acquires and transmits EEG data. As noted earlier, this technology is already in use to facilitate the early detection of drug efficacy.

New efficacy measures in trials

Given the broad range of physiological data that can be acquired through this technology, new and possibly more objective outcome measures can be incorporated into trial design. For example, in clinical trials that evaluate subjects with Parkinson's disease, attention deficit hyperactivity disorder (ADHD), and Alzheimer's disease, improvement is measured by clinician-rated instruments. Several issues can negatively impact clinician-rated evaluations: the clinical skill level and sophistication of the rater, the potential for bias and rater inflation, and the quality of rater training provided for the trial. A wireless actigraph sensor provides an opportunity to supplement traditional data sources with continuous information about the subjects' activity level. This type of data can provide insights into the efficacy of the study medication (Van Someren Eus et al., 2006).

Subject compliance and failed CNS trials

Increasingly, many therapeutic areas, including CNS, are experiencing increased placebo response and, more worrisome, failed trials. These problems stem from numerous factors related to the investigative site, the subject, or the design of the protocol. Subject non-compliance with study medication can also be an important cause of failed trials. Certainly, the most extreme case of medication non-compliance is seen with the professional patient who takes no study medication during the trial but reports good compliance and returns empty medication cards or bottles to the investigative site. Wireless sensor technology provides solutions to identify and actively intervene with poorly compliant subjects. Various emerging device companies offer solutions to monitor compliance remotely. One such company is Xhale, which can detect real-time study medication compliance. Subjects take the study medication and then, 10 minutes later, breathe into a breathalyzer-like device, allowing the detection of a taggant that had been added to the study medication or its capsule. Other technologies widely available allow the remote monitoring of the opening and closing of a medication bottle (e.g., GlowCaps device by Vitality).

Post-approval safety surveillance

Increasingly, the FDA has adopted a life-cycle approach to product development and evaluation. With the passage of the FDA Amendments Act 2007 (FDAAA Title VIII and IX), there is greater need for improved safety signal detection during development and post-approval of a compound (Kenkeremath, 2008). This legislation encourages the application of new information technology and tools to better understand the safety profile of the molecule. Since Phase IIIb and IV research programs tend to be more cost-sensitive than registration research, active surveillance via wireless sensor technology offers a solution to improve signal detection with little increase in variable costs.

Direct-to-patient trials

In June 2011, Pfizer and Mytrus announced the first all-electronic, home-based clinical trial of a drug, which was approved by the Food and Drug Administration (Dooren, 2011). The trial is designed to replicate the results of a previously done trial in overactive bladder disorder that was conducted by Pfizer in 2007 evaluating their drug Detrol compared to placebo. The electronic trial, called the REMOTE trial, will recruit participants through Internet advertisements and direct them to the study's website. On the website, patients will learn about the study and, if they qualify, enroll in the trial. The electronic study will require that patients have blood samples taken, which will be drawn at a local clinic or during a home visit. Medications will be mailed to patients. Outcome measures will be gathered through assessments accessed by participants on the study website. Participants will also keep diaries using a smart phone application that has been created for the trial.

This innovative approach to a completely remote or virtual trial brings obvious advantages over the traditional, site-based approach, where subjects are identified, enrolled, and data collected by investigative sites contracted to work on the trial. The key benefits of a remote trial relate to reducing overall trial costs through minimal trial infrastructure and having access to a far larger pool of research patients, who are not bound geographically to investigative sites. While REMOTE is a Phase IV trial, it is anticipated that success with this trial and other late-phase trials will prompt the various stakeholders to consider the use of direct-to-patient approaches for more Phase II/III trials.

New product development: moving beyond a pill

It is no longer sufficient for a pharmaceutical company just to receive a marketing license from a regulatory authority for a new drug – the drug has to be reimbursable. Third-party payers across the globe, whether public or private, are exerting greater control over market access to pharmaceuticals, basing decisions on not only the safety and efficacy of the drug but its relative efficacy compared to existing treatment options.

Public payers are solely responsible for reimbursement decisions in the European Union member states, Canada, Japan, and Australia, whereas in the United States, about 80% of the total amount spent on pharmaceuticals is covered by third-party payers, and, with the recent passage of legislation providing a drug benefit for Medicare recipients (i.e. Medicare Part D), the public's share of costs for pharmaceuticals in the USA is growing (Eichler et al., 2010).

Thus, with third-party payers picking up more of the tab for pharmaceutical costs, pharmaceutical companies now must be prepared to demonstrate the relative efficacy of their new products compared to existing therapies. Even drugs that have been successfully launched are coming under increased scrutiny of payers. Consider the highly publicized CATIE trial, where a first-generation antipsychotic was reported to have a similar efficacy and safety to various second-generation antipsychotics (Lieberman et al., 2005). Although the results of the CATIE trial have been debated in various scientific circles (Manschreck and Boshes, 2007), more comparative efficacy research is under way with results that may threaten current reimbursement schemes for patented drugs.

It's not hard to imagine that the pharmaceutical industry will continue to face strong headwinds in the years to come – the industry will need to demonstrate that their products deliver real and measurable value over existing therapies, particularly when compared to generic drugs. The challenge is very real. If the industry fails to meet the challenge, we can expect to continue to see significant market disruptions as other entities (perhaps competitors from emerging markets) will rise to fill the market void.

Transformation of the industry

Today, the value proposition offered by drug manufacturers for their new products involves therapeutic innovation, that is, for a premium price, the branded drug will provide some incremental improvement in efficacy over existing therapies. This value proposition will not protect the industry from disruptive market forces that will diminish profitability and precipitate more market turmoil.

What is the correct prescription for an ailing pharmaceutical industry?

The answer may lie in leveraging some of the technological advances that have already been discussed in this chapter. There exist today various technologies that can be integrated into the clinical drug development process that will decrease development costs. Regulatory authorities are aware of these developments, and so far have expressed a willingness to consider the new approaches. With the average cost of bringing a new drug to market in the USA reaching nearly $1 billion, new methods to reduce development costs are a necessity (Adams and Brantner, 2010).

Perhaps an equally important consideration is to imagine how a pharmaceutical product could be more valuable to patients and, ultimately, payers. What if drugs were combined or bundled with appropriate technologies to deliver a therapeutic benefit that greatly exceeds the incremental value of the drug alone?

For example, consider the widespread phenomenon that most patients do not take their medications as prescribed. Taking this thought experiment further, imagine a new antidepressant which is 10% more effective than the next best approved medication. This 10% improved therapeutic advantage is at risk of being completely undermined in real-world application, where patients on average take medications as prescribed only slightly more than half the time (Cramer and Rosenheck, 1998).

How can we drive innovation

It's pretty clear from literature that non-compliant or poorly compliant patients will have far worse health outcomes than compliant patients (Cramer and Rosenheck, 1998). In this instance, a significantly more innovative product could be offered if the new antidepressant were bundled with a surveillance and reminder system. Many different types of technologies exist today that could be used, e.g. the Proteus Biomedical ingestible chip, which is embedded on the antidepressant drug and detects medication compliance. The embedded chip will send a compliance signal when it comes in contact with the patient's stomach. The signal is sent via a gateway device such as a smart phone. When no signal is detected, the phone would be programmed to send a reminder text message to the patient or to a member of the patient's support system to encourage compliance.

As an alternative to the ingestible chip, several smart phone apps are available today that offer different daily medication reminder services to patients.

Innovation could be pushed further by monitoring the individual patient's ability to tolerate the medication. If our new antidepressant had the potential for postural hypotension, a smart patch, bundled with the pharmaceutical product, could detect whether an individual patient is tolerating the medication. Physiological data would be gathered from the smart patch placed on the patient's skin. Software analytics would alert healthcare providers and/or the patient when the data suggest a tolerability problem, allowing for a dose adjustment before problems could be seen clinically, such as the patient falling or becoming lightheaded. The combination of a drug bundled with a surveillance system for safety, tolerability and compliance would be a huge step forward in an attempt to manage health outcomes.

"Choose the harder right rather than the easier wrong"

At the US Military Academy at West Point, cadets learn the phrase, "choose the harder right rather than the easier wrong". For the industry, the harder right is to experiment with new models of clinical drug development and offer innovative products that demonstrate clear and substantial improvement in health outcomes. The work will not be easy, and technological problems will need to be solved and regulatory hurdles cleared. Of course, the easy road for the industry would be to continue to do what it has been doing for years, developing drugs that are similar to existing treatments or only marginally better – taking this road will practically guarantee its obsolescence.

References

Adams, C. P. and Brantner, V. V. (2010). Spending on new drug development. *Health Econ*, 19, 130–41.

Cramer, J. and Rosenheck, R. (1998). Compliance with medication regimens for mental and physical disorders. *Psychiatr Serv*, 49, 196–201.

Cutler, D. M. (2007). The demise of the blockbuster? *New Engl J Med*, 356, 13.

Dooren, J. C. (2011). A clinical drug trial via phone, computer. *Wall Street Journal*, http://online.wsj.com/article/ SB100014240527023044323045 76369840721708396.html.

Eichler, H. G., Blooechl-Daum, B., and Abadie, E. (2010). Relative efficacy of drugs: an emerging issue between regulatory agencies and third-party payers. *Nat Rev*, 9, 277–91.

Jack, A. (2009). Novartis chip to help ensure bitter pills are swallowed. *Financial Times*, 21 September.

Kenkeremath, N. (2008). Clinical research and drug safety provisions of the FDA Amendments Act of 2007: trends, opportunities and challenges. A report prepared for ACRO by Leading Edge Policy and Strategy, LLC, 8 August.

Lieberman, J. A., Stroup, S., and McEvoy, J. P. (2005). Effectiveness of antipsychotic drugs in patients with chronic schizophrenia. *New Engl J Med*, 353, 1209–23.

Manschreck, T. C. and Boshes, R. A. (2007). The CATIE schizophrenia trial: results, impact, controversy. *Harv Rev Psychiat*, Sep-Oct, 15 (5), 245–58.

Saxon, L. A. and Gilliam, R. (2010). Long-term outcome after ICD and CRT implantation and influence of remote device follow-up. The ALTITUDE Survival Study. *Circulation*, 122, 2359–67.

Van Someren Eus, J., *et al.* (2006). New actigraph for long-term tremor recording. *Movement Disord*, 21, 1136–43.

Index

Printed in the United States
by Baker & Taylor Publisher Services